HEALTH CARE REFORM
THAT MAKES SENSE

A Detailed Plan to Improve America's Health Care
System from the Country's Leading Health Care CEO

Alan B. Miller

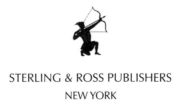

STERLING & ROSS PUBLISHERS
NEW YORK

Published by
Sterling & Ross Publishers
New York, NY 10001
www.sterlingandross.com

Paperback original.

Most Sterling & Ross books are available at special quantity discounts for bulk purchase for sales promotions, premiums, fund-raising and educational needs. Special books or book excerpts can be created to fit specific needs. For details, contact specialsales@sterlingandross.com

Library of Congress Cataloging-in-Publication Data

Miller, Alan B., 1937-
Health care reform that makes sense : a detailed plan to improve health care by America's leading health care CEO / by Alan B. Miller.
p. ; cm.
ISBN 978-0-9821392-9-5 (pbk.)
1. Health care reform--United States. I. Title.
[DNLM: 1. Health Care Reform--United States. 2. Insurance, Health--United States. 3. Models, Organizational--United States. WA 540 AA1 M547h 2009]
RA395.A3M765 2009
362.1'0425--dc22
2009041814

Contributing Editor: W.B. King
Book Design: Rachel Trusheim
Cover Design: Aritz Bermudez Monfort
©2009 Nederpelt Media

Printed in the United States of America
10 9 8 7 6 5 4 3 2 1

CONTENTS

1

AMERICAN HEALTH CARE:
THE ENVY OF THE WORLD

> Give me six hours to chop down a tree and
> I will spend the first four sharpening the axe.
>
> – ABRAHAM LINCOLN

IN ORDER TO ENGAGE in an insightful, progressive debate on the all-important issue of health care reform, the playing field must be leveled. The complexities are deep and far-reaching; however, logical options exist, many of which have not been included in the health care reform debates nor the current dilemma that has gripped the nation.

President Barack Obama presented a speech to a joint session of Congress on September 9, 2009. In it he said of the proposed health care reform bill, "There remain some significant details to be ironed out."

However well-intentioned the proposed health care reform bills are, Americans have been given the impression that politicians, especially in Washington, are empty suits taxing and spending. The proposed reform bill is dressed in a wrinkled suit and my iron is hot and steaming.

At one point during the president's speech, he promised not to sign a bill that would increase the deficit by one dime. With the proposed legislation costing nearly $1 trillion, can this be true? As a businessman, it seems to be an impossible premise. It is this flawed logic that has placed fear in the minds of many.

Americans are working hard to keep their respective heads above water during this recession. These are tough times and to many, health care reform is coming at them like a spinning curve ball.

In 1937, as the Great Depression was loosening its grip on the nation, I entered the world, landing in a blue-collar neighborhood in Brooklyn. My parents worked hard. Their focus was on making the rent each month and putting food on the table. They didn't have time to concern themselves with other pressing issues—life was about survival.

Many Americans today are faced with similar hurdles, especially when considering health care for themselves and their loved ones. I hold a high regard for hardworking Americans. As this charged debate began to unfold, I felt an ethical duty to share my experiences and insights.

TRANSPARENCY REQUIRED

The intricacies and issues surrounding health care are my specialty. My company, Universal Health Services, Inc., operates 137 private hospitals and allied facilities in the United States and Puerto Rico. As a result I'm uniquely positioned, and all too happy, to provide the average person with detailed knowledge on an otherwise overwhelming and subjective debate: what works, what doesn't, the hidden costs of existing programs like Medicare—the whole nine yards.

Everyday Americans have sounded off at town hall meetings across the country because they are confused and scared. And rightly so, as there is more misinformation than there is information.

In August 2009, as Congress was on recess fielding the increasing concerns from their constituents, a survey underwritten by AARP and conducted by Penn, Schoen and Berland Associates was released. Among its findings was that eight out of 10 Americans said they favored a "public option" insurance plan in national health care reform, but fewer than four out of 10 could correctly define what a public option meant. This is part and parcel of the problem. Understanding and defining key words and phraseology like *public option* or *single payer* will be covered further in subsequent chapters. I'll give you a hint though: the public option morphs into no option.

During the same time period, MSNBC released a poll that cited 94 percent of those surveyed felt there was a health care crisis, but of that number 77 percent said they had health insurance and were relatively happy with the coverage. The survey noted that in 2007, it was estimated that 85 percent of all Americans had some form of health insurance, which begs the question: is this really a crisis or a system in need of improvement?

No more smoke and mirrors. It's time to put politics and punditry aside and study the facts. Once knowledge is obtained and the public is informed, only then can a spirited conversation ensue. It is for this reason that after 30 years in the industry, I feel compelled to step forward.

I'm thankful for a rewarding career and a company that continues to build on a successful reputation. This book is for my children, my grandchildren and the generations of

Americans yet to come who deserve the opportunity to build on the promise of our forefathers. George Washington said the following during his Farewell Address to the American people, "Truth will ultimately prevail where there are pains taken to bring it to light."

FOCUS ON THE POSITIVE

There is no question that the current health care system has flaws. Essentially what we have is a vehicle that stalls periodically and has a rear tire slowly losing air. The idea is to address the engine trouble, perhaps a bad valve, and replace the tire, thus ensuring forward motion—a smoother ride with the American people in the driver's seat.

Our current health care system isn't a clunker, far from it. Upwards of 80 percent of the population is happy with the care they receive and don't want to see it compromised. Yes, the cost of premiums remains a concern to some and certain recommendations will be provided later in the book to cut unnecessary fat from procedural costs.

With that said, we have superior, world-class doctors, nurses and technicians who utilize state-of-the-art technologies in advanced hospitals. When one studies the medical care available in America with our capitalist system, it is fantastic—there is no parallel. Yes, there are inequities and there are inefficiencies, but these are the usual consequences associated with ventures of this magnitude.

A system built by humans will be impacted by human nature—some good and some bad. That's life. An adult, rational stance must be taken when considering our overall health care system. America leads the world in the medical industry because our system is based on incentive, risk and reward, which speaks to the very foundation of our country: entrepreneurship and hard work.

I celebrate what is right with our health care system and focus my energies toward fixing the inequities, which include insurance reform, tort reform, examining Medicare and Medicaid, analyzing the pervasive immigration issue and determining the actual number of uninsured Americans—a figure far less than the purported 45.7 million. The aforementioned topics will be covered in greater detail throughout the course of this book.

AVERT THE CRISIS

This health care debate is welcomed. The last time it became the talk at the watercooler was in 1993 under the Clinton administration. The fact that Americans are spirited, curious and engaged in the outcome represents a unique opportunity. Sixteen years ago, the pharmaceutical industry was not behind the reform. Today, they are interested in playing ball as long as contingencies are met.

For example, the current administration cut a tentative deal with the Pharmaceutical Research and Manufacturers of America (PhRMA). Over the next 10 years, PhRMA agreed to provide $80 billion of discounts to patients. In addition, it will spend approximately $150 million in advertising dollars to support the reform bill. In return, the administration agreed not to use its negotiating leverage to force unfair price cuts on the industry. Whether or not the deal will stand remains a big question.

We need to grab the reins and pull back so we don't

charge further into crisis mode. The stimulus package was presented, in a similar fashion to the current health care debate, as a crisis.

Our current administration signed off on a $787 billion bailout plan—that's a lot of zeros added to a smaller but significant bailout approved at the end of the previous administration. What happened? Not a whole lot; at least not yet, nor is there anything significant indicated on the horizon. Measured stimulation within an economic model is fine; it can help, but not at the levels our government has recently undertaken. The proposed health reform bill would be more of the same.

History is our teacher, and just as with the Great Depression and other market downturns, the economy eventually rights itself. Inventory is used up, prices go down far enough to attract business and people start buying again. Put simply, that's the cycle.

MEDICAL MARVELS

We need to put the brakes on and take a moment to focus on the most important aspects of our health care system: innovation and expertise. Not long ago, I heard a resident from one of the Caribbean islands say that if he has a headache, he takes an aspirin. If it is anything more severe, he calls his travel agent: he's heading to a hospital in Miami. He sounded like a smart man to me, and I'll tell you why.

We have the finest medicine in the world, with the finest doctors and the finest schools. If you take a look at international medical tourism—people with means and the ability to be discerning—you'll see an influx of foreigners taking advantage of our world-class medical services. Heads of state from the Arab nations on down the line go to the Mayo Clinic, the Cleveland Clinic, Memorial-Sloan Kettering, George Washington University Hospital and the list goes on.

I have operated hospitals in countries with socialized medicine, such as the United Kingdom and France. There is simply no comparison. This is not to say that there aren't excellent hospitals and doctors operating outside the United States. There are small pockets of reverse tourism in India and Singapore, for example, built largely on lowered prices, but overall, we remain the leaders. And for the most part, those doctors were educated in America.

We train countless Pakistani and Indian doctors, and when the majority of them complete their residency, they stay here. Leading reasons for this stronghold are that 70 percent of Nobel Prize recipients for medicine are from the United States. In addition, 77 percent of pharmaceutical advances take place in the United States and are then exported to other countries.

It is critical, however, to dig deeper than the numbers and statistics that become sound bites, fueling various arguments and stances on this highly volatile issue. Over the course of the last year, I have been the guest on countless radio and television news programs speaking on the pervasive issue of reform. Producers and on-air hosts are asking the right questions, but their three- to five-minute format simply doesn't provide enough time to adequately educate their viewers. This was yet another reason to write this book.

REFOCUS THE DEBATE

From the onset, the health care debate has gone down a number of distinct roads, the first of which was covering the uninsured. This concept was tied to the failing aspects of the economy. The rationale was that the cost of health care was an undue burden on the economy, and if these costs along with inflation couldn't be brought under control, then the economy could not be fixed.

These combined issues didn't gain as much traction as expected, which gave rise to the insurance reform issue. As with all systems, there is truth in that flaws exist. People often say, "I like my doctor but not my insurance company." Essentially, insurance companies became an easy target, and like all industries they should be subject to reform if the model is proven to be suspect.

As the various forms of the health care reform bill bounced around the House of Representatives and the U.S. Senate, it became unclear exactly which issue would be the selling point. A bill of this magnitude requires a handle for politicians to hold onto in order to support or reject it. Both sides of the aisle have made emotional arguments on behalf of their position, but more often than not there are factual inconsistencies that are reported in papers and magazines and then pushed through the mill, which is the 24-hour television and Internet news cycle. As a consequence, it becomes difficult for the American public to decipher what the facts are.

This is the nature of the political machine that is Capitol Hill. Perhaps the only flaw in our democratic system is the fact that presidential term limits influence policy initiatives.

Problems associated with health care have permeated the system for the last 40 or 50 years. And, theoretically, they should have been dealt with incrementally, issue by issue. Unfortunately, all too often the attitude is "not on my watch" and systemic problems are passed along.

The same could be said for corporations and businesses with CEOs who concentrate on quarter-to-quarter results. This places pressure on companies to be short-term oriented and to not focus on long-term investment. These companies, some of which were once household names, have failed. There is no guarantee that government programs, however well-intentioned, are not subject to the same fate. Who is left holding the bag? The American taxpayer will be the unwilling recipient of runaway costs and compromised health care. This is the reason we must proceed with caution.

There is no more time for an antiquated approach. In the beginning of 2009, when the health reform bills first were kicked around, Medicare was held up as a failing government program in need of change. By the end of the summer, it was being touted as a model for universal health care for all Americans. With misdirection and misinformation like this example, it is no wonder that people are confused.

The reality is that most Medicare recipients are satisfied, and in most cases happy, with their coverage. The problem is that it is a program that has wildly escalating costs and, according to some forecasts, is less than a decade away from bankruptcy. This is due to the fact that the program simply pays claims without vigorously investigating for fraud and abuse. In 2008, for example, Medicare's annual spending exceeded tax revenues, forcing Medicare to spend its reserve funds. To replicate the Medicare model for the rest of the country, or those deemed uninsured, seems incongruous.

I recently heard the story of a fine young doctor who went to work for the Veterans' Administration. He said he was pleased to be working with a group of people who were the most dedicated medical professionals he had yet to come across, that was, until four thirty in the afternoon. They punched the clock. They didn't stay a minute after their shift because they had zero incentive.

To be successful in business you accommodate to your customers' needs. The health care industry should be no different. This approach breeds excellence. Without incentive, there is little reward. And without drive, innovation is lost. The cascading result of this premise would be that highly educated doctors eager to help people would feel thwarted, disenchanted. Their once entrepreneurial profession will be considered a liability, and they may well turn their focus elsewhere, to another profession. A greater shame I cannot underscore.

RESPECT THE PROCESS

The balance of this book will investigate what is wrong with our health care system and ways in which it can be improved: diagnosis and remedy. As noted, the majority of my recommendations are not included in the various bills that were circulated during the writing of this book.

These are solutions I have discussed countless times over the years behind closed doors with peers, politicians, policymakers as well as the medical and insurance communities. It is now time to have the conversation with you, the

American people who deserve to see the issues from the inside out.

After all, health care represents 17 percent of our Gross Domestic Product (GDP). We simply can't afford any miscalculations. The *health* of our economy, and that of our people, depends on due diligence and foresight.

At this point everyone agrees that the "tree" should be trimmed, but as Abraham Lincoln said, let's spend more time sharpening the axe and less time chopping it down.

2

MEDICAL MALPRACTICE: A MALIGNANT TUMOR ON AMERICAN HEALTH CARE

Status quo is Latin for 'the mess we're in.'
— RONALD REAGAN

THE MALPRACTICE INDUSTRY represents $1 billion annually, which is a conservative estimate. Each year, Universal Health Services sets aside a reserve of approximately $75 million for fees associated with malpractice cases. It is the unfortunate price of doing business in our litigious society, which has severe rippling effects from operation and administration services on down to patient care. This is one of the biggest issues facing Americans today. As a result of the soaring number of malpractice cases, the delivery of quality health care may be impacted. Aside from agreeing to conduct "demonstration projects," the current administration has by and large left the issue of tort reform out of the health care reform debate, despite the fact that the nonpartisan Congressional Budget Office released a report in October 2009 that found that tort reform would cut the federal deficit upwards of $50 billion.

While Health and Human Services Secretary Kathleen Sebelius announced that the federal government would spend $25 million on pilot programs aimed at curbing malpractice lawsuits, it simply was a bone thrown to appease those opposed to the current health care reform bill that doesn't include real malpractice or tort reform. The minute amount of money that has been allocated is an indication that the administration has little interest in this fertile area for reform and cost reduction.

This dog and pony show approach is wrong. This administration tried to quickly push through health care legislation and failed. Now they have the attention of the American public and all the politicians who represent them. Instead of simply appeasing detractors, they should go back to the drawing board and offer sound solutions that address all issues and concerns, such as malpractice tort reform. However, logic and politics are words not often used in the same sentence. Putting it succinctly, Howard Dean, M.D., former chair of the Democratic Party, said in an answer to why liability reform is not in the proposed legislation, "The reason why tort reform is not in the bill is because the people who wrote it did not want to take on the trial lawyers in addition to everybody else they were taking on, and that is the plain and simple truth."

Universal Health Services recruits leading doctors to practice at our hospitals because we have state-of-the-art equipment, an extremely well-trained staff and a nursing team they can rely on. We spend a great deal of time and effort on risk management and controlling human error, an approach consistent with our business model: providing the highest quality care.

However, in any profession or calling, whether it is a police officer, lawyer, pilot or doctor, some mistakes will be made. Despite excellent care and the best intentions, as a company, we must be concerned with malpractice exposure and its effects.

FAIR COMPENSATION

There are two parts to a malpractice damage case: economic and noneconomic. If we operate under the assumption that something went wrong with a patient's procedure that was within the control of the physician or the hospital, then that patient was subject to malpractice and should be fairly compensated.

If, for example, a 37-year-old construction worker with two young children suffered a mistake in an operation that greatly hampered him from further pursuing his profession and lifestyle, economic damages can be assessed—how much he will lose in earnings. I support full compensation of economic damages. Nobody in my industry has a problem with this approach because it is reasonable, and from Universal Health Services' stance, it's the ethical and correct course of action.

The problem that emerges is part two of the malpractice platform: noneconomic damages otherwise known as pain and suffering. Economic damages are specifically quantified for the jury, such as the amount for medical bills or lost wages. Juries cannot award more in economic damages than the evidence supports. However, noneconomic damages are not quantified nor grounded by any financial or empirical foundation. These rulings lead to great abuse by trial lawyers. Despite the fact that all juries are instructed to not allow their sympathies sway verdicts, trial attorneys use noneconomic damages to prey upon juries' sympathies and obtain excessive jury awards that are often not based on logic or evidence. Current law prohibits trial attorneys or juries from using damages to "send a message" or "teach them a lesson." Trial attorneys, however, are accustomed to using noneconomic damages to subvert these prohibitions and increase jury awards through inflammatory appeals effectively turning noneconomic damages into punitive damages, which they are not.

When large settlements are handed down, monies are divided before the plaintiff receives his or her share. A *New England Journal of Medicine* study found that for every $1 awarded to a plaintiff in a malpractice suit, 54¢ went to lawyers, expert witnesses, courts and other administrative expenses.

Hypothetically speaking, let's say there is a situation involving an upcoming birth. The obstetrician/gynecologist (OB/GYN) has instructed the patient that due to her age and previous health issues, the delivery has been labeled "difficult." Protocol dictates that the OB/GYN check off a requirement sheet every 15 minutes during the labor and after birth. While many of these procedures are taped, if the defendant, or the hospital, can't prove that the doctor was attending to the patient at that exact moment of the incident or accident cited in the malpractice case, the fault often falls on the defendant.

There are many issues related to the doctors' documentation of medical procedures. Yes, in certain lawsuits the doctor is at fault, but all too often the doctor is doing his or her job dealing with what was already deemed a difficult delivery and simply did not have time to sign a checklist because he or she was involved in potentially life-saving measures. When these cases are tried before the court, lawyers comb the files looking for a technicality. The trial lawyer will invariably underscore that requirements weren't met, even if the doctor was doing his or her best on behalf the patient, but something still went wrong. This simply is not fair. If you're in the middle of a crisis and you have to stop and remember to sign off on a checklist, does that equate to the best possible medical care?

RATES CLIMB AND DOCTORS GO

There needs to be a cap on noneconomic damages so that runaway jury awards, out of proportion to the incidents, can be avoided. The previous administration attempted to pass tort reform through on the federal level, but in the end it stalled and the situation remained static, which gave trial lawyers continued cause for celebration.

The former editor of *The New England Journal of Medicine*, Dr. Arnold Relman, estimated that direct costs of malpractice litigation are approximately $7.5 billion annually. We are dealing with big numbers here. So what's the bottom line, the result of rampant malpractice cases? Insurance rates go through the roof, forcing well-meaning physicians to pay escalating premiums. In some cases, they restrict their practices while others relocate to one of the 28 states that have enacted reform that supports lower insurance premiums.

Medical Malpractice Rates for Florida (2007)

General Area	Internal Medicine	General Surgery	OB/GYN
Broward County	$54,074	$208,200	$213,533
Dade County	$54,450	$207,300	$238,000
Palm Beach County	$43,175	$161,400	$187,500
Remainder of state	$28,950	$108,700	$125,500

Source: Above figures are approximations across various carriers serving the FL malpractice liability mal market. Underlying data taken from the Medical Liability Monitor 2007 Rate Survey. The rates shown above should not be interpreted as the actual premiums an individual Florida physician pays for coverage. © 2008-2009 NJSave LLC. As shown on the Florida resource page of CoverMD.com: www.covermd.com/Resources/Florida_Medical_Malpractice_Insurance.aspx.

It's a hit-or-miss proposition for operators within the health care industry. For example, OB, orthopedics and neurosurgery are three specialties where perfect success rates are difficult to achieve. OBs are dealing with situations out of their control such as the mothers' approach to prenatal care, mothers' health issues and drug abusers, among other factors. People forget in this country, which is a good thing, that only 70 plus years ago mother and child mortality rates during delivery were significantly higher. Successful delivery is now routine! We've come a long way.

Americans want a perfect outcome when it comes to most things in their lives, including medical care. I don't blame them. There are many people living in Third World countries that are sick and continuously suffering. And whereas that was once the case in America, our superior health care system has relieved so many people of these hardships. This is yet another example that our medicine and facilities are superior, a result of an incentive-based healthcare system. Take that away, or force doctors into a corner where they can't practice without going broke, and the game will change. In many respects, I have seen the game change over the last 30 years.

In New York, where there is no cap on noneconomic damages, for example, physicians in specialties such as neurosurgery and obstetrics must pay $200,000 a year for malpractice coverage. New York is among the states in which my company does not operate. In 2008, the New York Public Interest Research Group released a federal data report where it found that for the past 15 years in New York, 2,000 to 2,400 malpractice claims were made each year, which altogether amounted to $743 million in payouts. Conversely, the state of Ohio passed tort reform in 2003 that capped noneconomic damages at $250,000 and punitive damages at $1 million. According to the Ohio Department of Insurance, in 2006 there were 4,006 medical malpractice claims reported compared with 5,051 in 2005, which represents a 20 percent decrease.

In other states, such as Pennsylvania, which has no cap, a state fund was created to supplement private malpractice coverage to retain and attract quality physicians. In the absence of a cap, doctors couldn't afford the high insurance premiums on their own and some left the state to practice elsewhere.

State Tort Reform

Type of Reform	# of States	Summary	States That Have Enacted the Reform
Modify Joint-and-Several Liability	38	States have based the amount for which a defedant can be held liable on the proportion of fault attributed; however, the formulas differ substantially from state to state. In addition, most of the reforms apply to specific types of torts or have other restrictions.	AK, AZ, AR, CA, CO, CT, FL, GA, HI, ID, IL, IA, KY, LA, MA, MI, MN, MS, MO, MT, NE, NV, NH, NJ, NM, NY, ND, OH, OR, PA, SD, TX, UT, VT, WA, WV, WI, WY
Modify the Collateral-Source Rule	25	Typical reforms either permit evidence of collateral-source payments to be admitted at trial, allow awards to plaintiffs to be offset by other payments, or both.	AL, AK, AZ, CO, CT, FL, GA*, HI, ID, IL, IN, IA, KS*, KY, ME, MI, MN, MO, MT, NJ, NY, ND, OH, OK, OR
Limit Noneconomic Damages	23	Punitive limits from $250,000 to $750,000. Note: More than half of the reforms apply to torts involving medical malpractice.	AL*, AK, CO, FL, HI, ID, IL*, KS, MD, MI, MN, MS, MT, NV, NH*, ND, OH, OK, OR*, TX, WA, WV*, WI
Limit Punitive Damages	34	Limitations include outright bans; fixed dollar caps ranging from $250,000 to $10 million; and caps equal to a multiple of compensatory awards.	AL, AK, AZ, AR, CA, CO, FL, GA, ID, IL*, IN, IA, KS, KY, LA, MN, MS, MO, MT, NE, NH, NJ, NY, NC, ND, OH, OK, OR, SC, SD, TX, UT, VA, WI

*The only relevant law enacted since 1986 was found to violate the state's constitution.
Source: Congressional Budget Office, *The Effects of Tort Reform: Evidence from the States* (June 2004).

DEFENSIVE MEDICINE

As a result of malpractice lawsuits driving up insurance rates, an unfortunate trend has occurred in the way in which doctors practice medicine—defensively! I don't blame them since they are working within the system that has been presented to them. They, too, are running a business.

DEFENSIVE MEDICINE

$100 billion cost per year.

Costs the average American family an additional $1,700 to $2,000 per year for health care.

Source: Stanford University (Daniel Kessler and Mark McClellan)

When I entered the health care industry, defensive medicine was not an issue for doctors. Let's say a patient came into an emergency room 30 years ago complaining of neck pain. If the conclusion was that it wasn't a life-threatening or serious issue, the patient was sent home with a couple tablets of painkillers and told to see his or her primary care doctor if problems persisted. A battery of tests would be ordered if the condition then warranted.

Today, that same scenario would play out much differently. The doctor would order expensive tests such as a CAT scan or an MRI. At the end of the day, for 99 percent of the cases, the diagnosis is the same: there is nothing seriously wrong. We see this scenario play out over and over again in our hospitals. It is an expensive cycle that continuously drives up the cost of care.

The practice of medicine has changed drastically. Today, so much of what doctors do in terms of treatment and prescription is done for legal reasons. In addition to acting in the patient's best interest, the doctor is concerned with how the medical record may be interpreted by a plaintiff's attorney two years down the road. This is one of the insidious results of the fear of malpractice lawsuits. These laws have placed both doctors and patients between a rock and a hard place.

A recent survey by the Massachusetts Medical Society and the University of Connecticut Health Center revealed that among physicians surveyed, 83 percent reported that they had practiced defensive medicine. That study showed that an average of 28 percent of tests, procedures, referrals and consultations were ordered for defensive reasons, for fear of lawsuits. The study also concluded that 13 percent of all hospitalizations may have been ordered by physicians for defensive purposes.

Such care is expensive as well as unnecessary. Overall, defensive medicine has been estimated to cost between $100 billion and $178 billion per year, according to a study by Daniel Kessler and Mark McClellan of Stanford University. That is an additional $1,700 to $2,000 paid every year by the average American family for unnecessary healthcare.

A 2005 American Medical Association survey found that 42 percent of doctors restricted their practices to avoid patients with complex medical problems and complicated procedures such as trauma surgery. When doctors' malpractice insurance rates significantly spiked in the beginning of this decade, the industry further fragmented. At this point, doctors began to build their own surgery and imaging centers in order to supplement their incomes to help offset rising insurance premiums.

Doctors make money by providing necessary services to patients. In some cases, this has resulted in the "selling" of procedures and screenings, which has further compromised the practice of medicine in the United States. If people want to talk about a crisis, they should look to excessive malpractice awards and its rippling effects.

LEGISLATIVE PROWESS

If there is a model to follow, we need to look west. In 1975, California's Medical Injury Compensation Reform Act was passed. As the legislation was being drafted, I traveled to California and spoke publicly in support of the bill while CEO of my first company, American Medicorp.

I'm not late to this party; I have fought long and hard for the passage of legislation that limits noneconomic damage awards on a national level. For the last 30 years it has been a state-by-state fight and there are still 22 states to go.

The California law was groundbreaking and encouraging in that to this day it limits noneconomic damages to $250,000, restricts lawyers' fees, requires that juries be notified if a malpractice victim has health insurance or another source of compensation and requires that malpractice defendants be notified of a pending lawsuit in a reasonable time to present a defense.

For an OB, the insurance rate in California is approximately $65,000 for malpractice insurance, whereas in New York it is more than double that amount. If you were in that profession where would you want to work? In Pennsylvania there are leading medical universities, but it is harder and harder to find an OB for the same reason; high insurance rates.

Is it a perfect system? The answer is no. California took a step in the right direction, but there is a long way to go. Among my recommendations to be covered in subsequent chapters will be a federally mandated program that uses California, as well as the many states that followed suit, as the model.

PERSEVERE: A PERSONAL REFLECTION ON HEALTH CARE

I'm a tall guy at six feet five inches. Basketball is my sport. I played in high school, was scouted and ultimately secured a full scholarship to the University of Utah, which at the time was ranked number three in the country. Before I agreed, the head coach took my mother and me to a nice dinner in Manhattan. I was just 16 years old and it all seemed glamorous. I sort of knew where Utah was, but I didn't really know where I was going. I just knew I wanted to leave Crown Heights, Brooklyn.

I spent nearly a year at the University of Utah before transferring on another full scholarship—sight unseen— to my alma mater, the College of William & Mary, where I played as a forward for the Tribe.

Athletics taught me the importance of teamwork and working hard because the more you put into something the more you get out of it, which is the approach I have used in my business pursuits. Basketball taught me in many ways to never give up and that good things tend to happen when you persevere.

Another lesson athletics taught me was to deal with adversity, which came in handy in 1957 during my second year on the team. I had redshirted my first year to save a year of eligibility. On a snowy winter night at the beginning of the season, my team was on route to the University of Pennsylvania in two station wagons: old Fords with wood paneling on the sides.

We had stopped off Route 301 in Maryland to have dinner. These were the days before the Turnpike. As we finished up, I walked outside as it started to snow harder. We got on the road and the snow continued to fall. We reached a top of a hill and I remember seeing four headlights coming at us. I can still recall watching this car heading straight for us in the wrong lane. In my head I said, "Whoa, they are going to hit us," but no words came from my mouth. I didn't look away or duck.

In those days, station wagons had three bench seats. On top of the seat was a steel bar to hold on to—like a bus. On impact, my head slammed down on the bar. The bar was tougher than I was—that was the end of my face. My nose was severely broken. I had a slight fracture to my skull from the impact on my forehead. It was a bloody mess.

I spent a month in a Washington, D.C. hospital where I received several operations to reconstruct my face. As I healed from each operation, another would be scheduled. In total, I would have six surgeries. The doctor was great. I still remember his name: William Carey Melloy. He literally attached a wire to my face during surgery and pulled it up because my face was depressed. I received terrific treatment. He said it was my strong bones that saved my life. I took a beating but survived and made a full recovery.

The college paid for my hospital stay and all related surgeries and care. There weren't as many lawsuits in those days. A lawyer did approach us as an action was taken out against the other car who hit us. The drivers were unemployed hockey players from Canada en route to Florida. Nothing materialized, although all six of us riding in that second wagon sustained severe injuries such as a punctured lung and a broken leg. But I was the big winner that day.

I wasn't able to play basketball again with the Tribe, which was a devastating blow. I worked my whole life for the opportunity to play college basketball. I had no aspirations past college but knew that I was cut short of a promising college career.

As I deal with health care issues, I come to the table with empathy because I've been the guy in the severe accident; the guy in the hospital bed dependent on the health care system. I am thankful to have had a positive experience.

I do my best to translate my personal experience to my business model: provide patients with excellent health care and move them along so they can get on with their lives.

THE PHARMACEUTICAL DEBATE

The health care system is comprised of many components. Among them is the pharmaceutical industry, which is essential to overall treatment success rates. While some might feel it is an industry that enjoys excessive profits, on the whole, an extraordinary amount of groundbreaking work has been accomplished, thus saving millions of lives. In 2008, 3.5 billion prescriptions were filled in the United States.

There is a significant difference in medicine and health care today versus 20, 30 or 50 years ago, which is due, in part, to the growth and life-saving research of the pharmaceutical industry. As I noted in chapter one, 77 percent of pharmaceutical innovation takes place in the United States. The positive benefits to these developments are hard to quantify because they are tremendously far-reaching. Take cancer survival rates, for example.

People often will ask: why does this drug cost what it costs? The short answer: there might be $100 million and eight to 10 years of hard work behind that drug. During that period of research, development and waiting for Food and Drug Administration (FDA) approval, the company did not make a cent. The average American would be surprised how many drugs are not approved and the amount of investment that was lost. Business is about taking chances, in hopes of an appropriate reward.

If the company is fortunate to receive FDA approval for a drug and is able to bring the product to market, they only have 17 years under a U.S. patent to recoup investments and make a well-deserved profit. Is that fair to the company?

What happens to the profit? These are usually publicly traded companies. The profit goes back into the company. Sure, it pays the executives, the managers and the scientists, it may pay a dividend, but the balance is put back into research and development and the process begins again.

Profits from medical technologies and advancements aren't hoarded or buried in a hole; they are recirculated throughout our society in various ways. These companies invest in innovation. Since it is not in their everyday purview, people outside the industry do not normally understand how these systems operate.

Inevitably, when a product does come to the market, the consumer might ask: how can a pill cost $100 (or whatever the price may be)? On average, people don't understand this process. In large part, it is our political and business leaders who have the responsibility to inform. In order to have forward motion on critical issues surrounding health care reform, a sense of transparency must exist. This is not to say that everyone will agree with what they learn, but profiting from advancements in medicine is not to be looked down upon. Nor is the profit generated through the work of often tens of thousands of talented people.

A business that competes for customers will always do a good job of servicing them and responding to their needs. We wouldn't have technological advancements such as the iPhone, for example, if the government was in charge of the cellular phone market. Apple created the iPhone because there is a need for it, and they did their part by investing in an innovation that spurred technological growth. In response, Blackberry, Motorola and a host of other companies continue to invest and explore new technologies in an attempt to gain market share. This is the American way of doing business.

We associate growth and innovation with private enterprise. We don't associate it with large government enterprises. Why? The reason is the government doesn't provide incentives for innovation or risk taking.

EDUCATION, INSIGHT AND OVERSIGHT

It never ceases to amaze me that in this country "profit" is a dirty word to some. One of the reasons is that we no longer teach enough economics and about our capitalistic system in our schools. For some reason, "nonprofit" is a good thing. "For profit" is deemed to be negative.

I have contributed to different educational platforms, including the Pennsylvania Economy League. This organization partners with government, business and civic groups to develop consensus and action on programs that can increase the effectiveness of state and local governments striving to improve Pennsylvania's economic competitiveness.

An exciting aspect of the program, which I fully support, brings area high school students together and educates them on various economic issues. Children today are not taught enough about the principles of capitalism and the great standard of living it has provided. The vision of those great men who founded this country was based on freedom and opportunity. If a stand is not taken to uphold these fundamental principals, we face an uncertain future. Alexander Hamilton said, "Those who stand for nothing fall for anything." I stand for capitalism and support an incentive-based private sector.

The pharmaceutical industry has, in certain respects, flourished but was deemed by some to make an unreasonable profit margin. Yet, the industry represents just 2 percent of our overall economy. A lack of education feeds this misunderstanding for many Americans who are trying to understand the various components of the health care industry.

There seems to be a growing number of Americans who do not hold business and enterprise in high regard. If we trace the steps back to the classroom, we know that business principles are not leading components of curricula. Most teachers are not overly compensated. An equally important profession like journalism also doesn't pay a lot of money.

As a result, a bias can exist against highly competitive business professionals who are well compensated. Academics may believe that they are smarter than the average person in general because they invested in their education and in turn themselves. If they are earning $63,000 per year and a peer who got lucky with an invention makes hundreds of thousands of dollars per year, they can become envious. It's human nature.

In a way, the system does not seem fair to some, but this is the capitalistic system our country was founded on. I support teachers getting paid more because their job is critical to the future of the nation, but they also have to understand that their position is risk-free and secure, whereas an entrepreneur's is unsecure and based on risk. As a result, certain teachers and journalists unwillingly, perhaps subconsciously, insinuate these biases into the educational system and the media.

On occasion, a pharmaceutical company will do the wrong thing. They get doctors to endorse a product, creating a conflict of interest. Recently, Pfizer, Inc. agreed to pay

$2.3 billion to settle charges that it illegally marketed the pain drug, Bextra, and three other medicines for uses that weren't approved by the FDA. In my hospitals, the doctors are independent and bring in their own patients; if they were to go on to endorse a product, we wouldn't necessarily know or have any control over it. Rather, the oversight comes from various medical societies such as the American Medical Association.

Again, is the system perfect? The answer is no. A system of checks and balances exists that can and should be applied to all aspects of health care. This approach will serve to address problems such as rampant malpractice cases or pharmaceutical companies that have done wrong, but it shouldn't cast a dark shadow over the whole debate. There are far more good things happening with American health care than there are bad.

MAYO CLINIC MODEL

During a speech in Minneapolis in September 2009, President Obama said, "Look at what the Mayo Clinic is able to do. It's got the best quality and the lowest cost of just about any system in the country. So what we want to do is we want to help the whole country learn from what Mayo is doing... That will save everybody money."

This approach is somewhat oversimplified. The Mayo Clinic and the Cleveland Clinic is a conglomeration of highly trained and highly qualified physicians. People go to these clinics from literally all over the world to seek the best medical care. The argument has been made that the federal system should emulate these clinic models because they make money and offer superior treatment. The Mayo Clinic's revenues are approximately $9 billion annually and approximately 250 surgeries are performed each day.

The clinic employs 3,300 physicians, scientists and researchers and 46,000 allied health staff workers at its three locations, which include Jacksonville, Florida and Scottsdale/Phoenix, Arizona. In total, over 1 million patients are treated each year. Rochester, Minnesota, where the flagship clinic is located, doesn't have a large population of indigent patients or uninsured patients that we have in any one of our hospitals, or in other markets such as large metropolitan cities like New York and Los Angeles. The city has a population of 85,000 residents. The competition is Olmstead Medical Center, with 29 percent of patients receiving Medicaid. Conversely, only 5 percent of the Mayo Clinic's patients are covered under Medicaid.

A 2005 study of federal employee insurance by the Government Accountability Office found that the Mayo Clinic charges among the highest rates for those people paying out of pocket for services. These include a majority of foreigners.

While the Mayo Clinic supports elements of the reform bill, it is opposed to a government-run insurance plan, or public option. In a letter to the Senate Finance Committee on September 15, 2009, the Mayo Clinic's Executive Director Jeffrey O. Korsmo wrote, "If the 'public plan' means a government-run, price-controlled, Medicare-like insurance model, we do not support it because it has been shown over many years that such a model has not controlled costs and has punished doctors, hospitals and others that provide high-quality, affordable care."

The Mayo Clinic model is based on the premise of it founders, Charles and William Mayo, whose philosophy was doctors should work on salary. There is an emphasis on cost-effectiveness with regard to patient care.

While incentives are critical to innovation, a problem emerges: providers are incentivized by the compensation-based procedures performed, such as surgeries, exams, tests or whatever the case may be. Often, these may be unnecessary and ultimately do not focus on maintaining a patient's wellness.

Some contend that providers should be paid for keeping patients healthy. We have seen capitated plans in California where doctors are paid a flat fee per patient. These doctors are encouraged to tailor a patient's treatment plan so that it supports a wellness program. It is in their interest to keep the patient healthy. So, there is merit in revisiting the incentive-based system in terms of patient care, but it is not a black-and-white issue.

These are the issues that can be explored so that common-sense solutions can be introduced into the current health care system. This requires cross-industry negotiation and teamwork, as well as limited input from the government.

If a new approach is not explored, the system remains fractured. Sensible solutions exist from those on the front line—hospital administrators and doctors. Ronald Reagan's take on the "status quo" is exactly right. We have a mess when it comes to the health care debate. We as a people are charged with the task of cleaning it up, and that concerted effort should not be left to government alone.

3

MEDICARE:
THE WRONG MODEL

Figures don't lie, but liars figure.

– MARK TWAIN

SAMUEL CLEMENS, under the famous pen name of Mark Twain, wrote the above line many years ago, but it still rings true. In business, I see this adage come to pass often, but at the end of the day, it is aggregated hard facts that support the bottom line.

Among the issues surrounding the health care reform debate that I find troubling is the purported 45.7 million, or 15.3 percent, of Americans who are classified as uninsured.

The aforementioned statistic came from a 2007 Department of Labor survey that was done in conjunction with the Census Bureau. Due to the recession and the rising unemployment rate, many analysts feel this number has grown by more than two million. Often pundits will round up this figure to 48 million.

When people hear this statistic on television or read about it in the papers, they are given the impression that 48 million sick, sad sacks are sitting around the country without insurance coverage and that it is a disgrace to America.

Americans, by and large good-hearted people, say, "We cannot have that, not in the wealthiest, most powerful country in the world." These statistics are wrong, yet are used to incite a sense of crisis.

During the president's joint address to Congress, he backed away from the aforementioned statistics and said that 30 million were uninsured. This certainly implies the purported number of uninsured is not only inaccurate but far lower than initially discussed.

GOOD INTENTIONS GONE AWRY

In 1945, during an address to the nation, President Harry Truman said:

> "Millions of our citizens do not now have a full measure of opportunity to achieve and to enjoy good health. Millions do not now have protection or security against the economic effects of sickness. And the time has now arrived for action to help them attain that opportunity and to help them get that protection."

Twenty years would pass before his thought came to fruition. On July 30, 1965, President Lyndon Johnson headed to the Truman Library located in Independence, Missouri to sign the Medicare and Medicaid programs into law. President Truman sat at Johnson's side. Upon signing the bill, President Johnson said:

> "There are more than 18 million Americans over the age of 65. Most of them have low incomes. Most of them are threatened by illness and medical expenses that they cannot afford. And through this

new law, Mr. President, every citizen will be able, in his productive years when he is earning, to insure himself against the ravages of illness in his old age. This insurance will help pay for care in hospitals, in skilled nursing homes, or in the home. And under a separate plan it will help meet the fees of the doctors."

At the ceremony, President Truman became the first American to be signed up for Medicare. Obviously, the intent to provide health care for America's senior citizens is an admirable and just cause, but without a viable economic model, in the long run as much harm as good is created.

While these programs have serviced millions of Americans over the last 40 plus years, costs continue to escalate. The problem is only getting worse with no tourniquet in sight.

In 1965, there were 18 million Americans over the age of 65. In 2006, this demographic doubled to approximately 37 million people, or 12 percent of the population. With baby boomers reaching retirement age in 2011, it is estimated that 20 percent or 70 million people will be eligible for Medicare.

Currently, Medicare receives roughly 11 percent of federal non-entitlement tax dollars. Estimates are that by 2020, this will be one in every five tax dollars, and by 2030, one in every three dollars. By 2050, it is estimated that one in every two tax dollars will go toward Medicare. This will be the situation if there is no change to the current model.

What happens if reform adds those aged less than 65 years to Medicare?

FIGURING OUT THE LIE

The Emergency Medical Treatment and Active Labor Act of 1986 requires that participating hospitals—those that accept payment from the Department of Health and Human Services, Centers for Medicare and Medicaid Services (CMS) under the Medicare program—provide services to anyone needing emergency treatment regardless of citizenship, legal status or ability to pay.

The passage of this bill was due in part to "patient dumping," a past practice of hospitals refusing to treat people due to the inability to pay, insufficient insurance coverage, or the transferring of emergency patients because of forecasted high treatment costs.

The law applies to basically all hospitals with the exception of the Shriners Hospitals for Children, Indian Health Service hospitals and Veterans Affairs hospitals. For the balance of operators, this is basically an unfunded mandate that places a significant burden on the already tough task of operating a hospital successfully.

These "uninsured" Americans are in fact receiving world-class medical care. Often, the procedures and testing provided comes at great expense. Who gets left holding the bag: the government? The answer (which may be surprising to some) is, hospitals, again and again, year after year.

Universal Health Services' 2008 financial statements, for example, reflected a total of almost $1.1 billion in bad debts, charity care and uninsured discounts, representing the total of billed charges that went unpaid by patients. When our costs rise, we obviously make less money. Bad debt is an expense not unlike a utility bill. If this huge expense went away because every person would be required to be covered by an insurance policy, we would be better off. But if the insurance companies have to pay more to UHS, for example, they will raise premiums. The lines get blurry, and this is not a case of connect the dots. The bottom line is that the uninsured drive costs up. Is this fair?

I contend that there are approximately 16 to 18 million uninsured. This is where the focus of the debate should be instead of presenting an inflated number to the public that takes the spotlight off the issue of dealing with the real problems, which in part are mismanaged government programs.

My concern is identifying the people who require health care but slip through the cracks of a broken system. To find out who these people are, we need to differentiate between the "uninsured" and those who do not have access to heath care.

Taking a closer look, there are approximately 11 million people who qualify for government programs but do not apply. In our hospitals, we see this scenario all the time.

Patients come in without any insurance but are in need of treatment. We have protocol in place and begin to ask specific questions about their financial condition. Eventually we come to the realization that they are eligible for Medicare, Medicaid, or if the patient is a child, the State Children's Health Insurance Program (SCHIP). We facilitate the process and assist them in signing up and gaining coverage.

THE COVERAGE COVER-UP

If they are eligible, then why don't they participate? This is usually the next logical question and a good one to ask. Preexisting medical conditions do not exclude participation, so that is not a consideration.

Medicare, for example, has four categories: Part A, which is hospital insurance; Part B, which is medical insurance; Part C, which is essentially the combination of Part A and Part B with the main difference being that it is provided through private insurance companies approved by Medicare; and Part D, which is a stand-alone prescription drug coverage insurance. The majority of enrollees pay a premium for this coverage; however, plans and cost vary with options on drug plans.

Let's focus first on the ramifications Part A and Part B have on the health care free-form debate.

The majority of those who qualify receive Part A automatically when they turn the age of 65. This demographic doesn't have to pay a monthly payment or a premium because they or a spouse paid Medicare taxes while they were working. According to the Centers for Medicare & Medicaid Services, if they are not eligible for the premium-free option, they can pay up to $443 each month.

Part B of the Medicare plan has the majority of participants paying $96.40 per month, according to the U.S. Department of Health and Human Services. Certain people pay higher monthly premiums based on their modified adjusted gross income.

In essence, we have a portion of the population counted as uninsured who are essentially covered by insurance at all times, but wait until they need care and are forced to sign up. These people are skirting the system by not paying and driving up the costs of medical procedures and insurance premiums.

With Medicare alone, we have removed a significant percentage of the uninsured off the inflated figure of 45.7 million. Next we take a look at Medicaid, which is a federally mandated program that is managed by the state. Rules and requirements vary.

On average, citizens who are considered at the poverty level ($22,000 annual income for a family of four) are covered under the program. Components of the recent health care reform bill would raise the poverty level for eligibility to $88,000 for a family of four, which would severely damage an already failing system.

It is this approach that burdens the nation's ability to actually develop sound alternatives to health care reform. Until the conversation is changed, these types of suggested alternatives will be thrown into the mix, muddying the waters and clouding the view of existing problems.

There are other criteria for eligibility such as age, citizenship and disability. Additionally, certain states have programs that cater to those individuals who don't qualify for Medicaid. These programs are not federally funded.

ILLEGAL IMMIGRATION: ACCESS TO HEALTH CARE

Eligibility for children is not dependent on parent's citizenship status, which leads to the overarching, pervasive and expensive immigration issue. There remains a significant number—approximately 9.7 million—illegal or undocumented aliens. I don't think anyone is suggesting that this population of the "uninsured" be formally covered in any reform bill. Yet due to poor government oversight, loopholes exist and the system is being exploited.

Joe Wilson, the GOP congressman from South Carolina, became the story himself after President Obama addressed the joint session of Congress on September 9, 2009. While Obama said the reform bill wouldn't cover illegal immigrants, Wilson shouted, "You lie!"

While Wilson rightfully apologized to the president for his "inappropriate and regrettable" comments, the historical outburst mirrored in many ways the tenure of heated town hall meetings. The majority of attendees were seeking answers to proposed policies that the president admitted needed to be ironed out. For example, a provision that required a person to prove citizenship to receive government-funded health benefits was removed from the bill.

The American Council for Immigration Reform conducted a poll of 1,000 voters nationwide in August 2009. The survey found that 78 percent of Americans believe that high immigration levels have had an adverse impact on the quality and cost of our health care system. And while people claim this is a partisan issue, 89 percent of respondents were Republican and 69 percent were Democrats. This presents a clear majority in favor of immigration reform.

UHS operates a number of hospitals along the border in the southwest. We are adjacent to a significant immigrant population, which is a convenience for expectant mothers. Most are only a few miles away from our hospitals, but some drive a great distance to get close to the border. They wait until they are about to deliver, then drive across the border and present themselves at the emergency room. We take them in and facilitate the birth. If there are complications, we provide them with neonatal care or whatever care the child might require—an expensive proposition. All expenses associated with the child's care become the responsibility of the hospital.

In Texas, for example, the Harris County Hospital District treated over 26,000 illegal immigrants in 2008. This cost taxpayers $156 million. In total, the illegal immigration health care issue represents 12 percent of the county's $1.3 billion budget.

The consequence for hospitals is that defensive care comes into play. Since hospitals in certain markets understand that they will lose money due to this demographic, they calculate ways in which to lose the least amount of money. For example, if a pregnant woman enters the emergency room and is determined to be unhealthy, the hospital administrator is better off spending a hundred or thousands of dollars on prenatal care. The alternative is spending perhaps half a million dollars, when her baby is sick and needs to be treated in intensive care.

THE INVINCIBLE

According to a survey of colleges and universities by Aetna, Inc., there are approximately 4.7 million uninsured students. There is a remaining demographic, an estimated 9.1 million, who make upwards of $75,000 and choose not to buy insurance usually due to being in the 18 to 34 age demographic.

This group of uninsured feels invincible, adopting the "nothing can hurt me" stance. Even after my car accident at age 20, I still felt invincible because if that didn't kill me, I reasoned, what could? Now I'm older and know better. I understand the thought process these young people have, but not having insurance impacts health care costs and insurance premiums for others.

There is yet another sliver of the population between jobs or having recently accepted a new position who are waiting for their paperwork—their coverage—to kick in. Additionally, there are those unemployed on the Cobra plan (extended insurance coverage), which lasts 18 months. All totaled, this demographic is hard to quantify because it is ever changing—a revolving door.

A recent poll by United Health Group found that misinformation and lack of information also accounts for low insurance rates in the 18 to 34 age demographic. The company administered an online poll of 1,000 students ages 18 to 21. Eighty-two percent said the issue of health insurance was a necessity although 67 percent said they had not made any plans for health insurance coverage after graduation.

Why is there a problem? The study found that 69 percent of those currently covered by their parents' health insurance plans had little or no information on the policy's specifics. Twenty-six percent were not sure when their policy would be terminated. Eighty-seven percent polled said educators and educational institutions could and should do more to educate on topics associated with health insurance.

THE "UNINSURED"

Now, if we combine all of the above, we can deduct 27.7 million from the "uninsured" number of 45.7 million, which leaves us with approximately 18 million actually uninsured. The figure fluctuates by a few million because many in the system, such as those in between jobs, have a revolving door status.

In my estimation, there are ways to tackle these demographics and ensure they receive coverage. Turning the entire system upside down doesn't make sense. What does make sense is addressing existing, unsuccessful governmental programs that force the private sector to make up the difference.

Since existing government sponsored and operated health care programs have not been proven financially viable, why move forward with an estimated $1 trillion reform bill before addressing the root problems?

Taking a closer look, the administration's proposed cost for health care reform was initially $1.2 trillion. Due to the American public's sticker shock, the figure dropped to $1 trillion. In an attempt to present a more palatable figure to the American public, the Senate Finance Committee, in association with Congressional Budget Office, approved a reform bill in October 2009 that was scored at $829 billion, the theoretical cost to taxpayers. I used to be in the advertising business and this is known as psychological pricing. Obama further promised that the proposed health care reform wouldn't add "one dime" to the nation's deficit. It raises serious fiscal questions for the president to say that the money needed to support the reform bill will be found in part within the Medicare and Medicaid model, which in his words is "full of waste and abuse." The government has never been able to control such waste. In the end, it comes down to a sound business plan, which has yet to be presented.

MEDICARE FACTS

Medicare accounts for 14% of the Federal Budget.

In 1965, approximately 17 million were eligible.

Between 2010 and 2030, the number of people on Medicare is projected to rise from 46 million to 78 million.

Source: Medicare Payment Advisory Commission analysis of plan bid data from CMS, Nov 2007.

It is not an issue of *not* providing medical care to those in need, but rather approaching it in such a manner that the country, and its health care system, won't buckle and break under the pressure. It's a naïve approach to load the back of the donkey until it drops dead. This is exactly what is happening: incurring high levels of additional debt and taxation negatively impacts the economic strength of the nation.

I recognize there are many problems associated with health care from the cost of premiums to the ability to secure coverage from existing plans. These issues will be addressed in coming chapters. My approach is to identify all the variables of what is wrong first, and then go about the task of making my recommendations.

LOST IN THE SHUFFLE

While there are bright, well-intentioned men and women employed in various sectors of government, *bureaucracy,* by its nature, has the capacity to breed complacency because the model lacks incentive. As a consequence, there are many situations where those entitled to government-funded programs are turned down in the application process.

In some cases it takes more than one attempt to get signed up for available services. If an applicant is poorly educated or without the required knowledge to navigate the system, then that person, who theoretically should be covered by a government-sponsored health care program, is left on the sidelines.

If the system worked like a well-oiled machine, the health care debate would be far less complicated. The truth is, the federal government hasn't gotten it right, and it has had countless years to do so. In the private sector, it would have failed due to better competitors. The capable survive, others do not.

Take a look at the airline industry. Trans Worlds Airlines (TWA) was acquired by American Airlines in 2001. This company, once a household name, ultimately failed due to management mistakes that didn't allow the company to keep up with market pressures. The same philosophy doesn't apply to the government. If a government program fails, often they receive more money. This is a recipe for disaster.

We can look to states that tried to implement healthcare plans and also failed. Tennessee, for example, implemented managed care in the Medicare program in 1994. It was labeled TennCare. The idea was to use savings from Medicaid to cover children and the uninsured. Again, a well-meaning program, but in a few short years, it just about bankrupted the state and reduced the quality of health care.

TennCare was essentially a public option. By 1998, the program serviced 1.2 million residents. By the time the plan was reconstructed in 2006, the price tag had gone from $2.5 billion in 1995 to $8 billion. The state was forced to raise taxes to support the system. The reconstruction eliminated two segments of the program—TennCare Spenddown and Medically Eligible-Uninsurable—which represented approximately 170,000 residents.

One reason for the spike of participation in TennCare was that private businesses dropped health insurance for employees. This population migrated to the state plan. To this end, studies indicate that only 55 percent of TennCare recipients came from the uninsured population.

Along with residents cut from the program, so were benefits. This is a typical scenario. Those in favor of government-managed health care promise the moon in terms of what will be available to patients. When the costs are aggregated, however, it is a different story.

Then it becomes a matter of what the government can afford and often it cannot provide the best health care. This is yet another reason many Americans are wary of a public option. Many Tennessee doctors said they were overburdened by the bureaucratic system, which monopolized their time. In addition, doctors and hospitals weren't being fairly reimbursed for their services. As a consequence, physicians began to decline TennCare patients. In effect, those enrolled in the program had supposed benefits, but they were not guaranteed care.

As TennCare continues to flounder, the initial goal of providing health care is still not achieved. Instead, the state has lost a significant amount of money and still hasn't addressed the entire uninsured population.

Since it is a government-run program, it can't close its doors like TWA did. Rather, it will keep moving forward, losing money and not achieving the objective. Imagine if this model was applied to all 50 states? Keep in mind that Tennessee's population is approximately 6 million. As of July 2008, census data estimated the United States population at approximately 304 million. Imagine the impact of a single-payer system on a scale this large.

LEARNING THE ROPES

When President Obama told the joint session of Congress on September 9, 2009 that, "There remain some significant details to be ironed out," it hit home on many levels. I'm an only child and the grandson of Russian immigrants. My father, Manuel, owned a dry cleaning store. My father struggled, eventually lost his business and ended up working in a factory. My mother, Mary, a strong-willed woman, was a union organizer during the 1920s. She, along with my father, taught me the importance of hard work for which I'm forever grateful.

On weekends I had two jobs, one of which was delivering groceries from the local market. I always knew the cheap customers because after climbing six flights of stairs they would yell, "Just leave the bags at the door." No tip, zero; really nice.

I used my bicycle for that job as well as for my second job, delivering telegrams for Western Union—rain or shine. I would be paid 10¢ per delivered telegram. My best days were when I was sent to one of the local halls where receptions would be held after weddings and events of that nature.

For whatever reason, if people couldn't make the party, then they would send congratulatory telegrams. These were my most profitable days because I would deliver them in bundles, sometimes 20 at a time. That was a real prize of a day. Aunt Sophie from Cincinnati couldn't make it but sent her love—these sorts of messages. Lots of "God bless you" telegrams, wishing the couple well on their marriage.

I learned the importance of a good work ethic, which translated to my education. Being bright, I was placed in the Special Progress Program, which combined junior high school into a two-year program instead of three. Then I attended Thomas Jefferson High School (which isn't there anymore) where we won the city basketball championship in 1954. This remains one of my fondest memories. Four of the six key players on that team are still alive and I keep in touch with them. The experiences we shared on court I've kept with me all these years. I graduated from high school at 16 and headed off to the University of Utah.

I'm a student of history and an autograph collector, concentrating on U.S. presidents and generals who were leaders during tough times. Among my favorites are George Washington, Abraham Lincoln, General and President Dwight Eisenhower, General Norman Schwarzkopf, Civil War General John Fulton Reynolds and General Robert E. Lee who said, "Do your duty in all things, you can't do more and you should never wish to do less." In relation to the health care reform debate before us, Lee's quote is appropriate.

From politicians to business owners to the average American looking for answers, we must each do our respective duty. For me, this includes sharing my experiences and insights in hopes of providing more answers than questions.

There is a great lesson to be learned from our military. I have the highest regard for the military and our military academies—particularly the character of the officers. These men and woman are among the finest people in our nation. Their willingness to give their lives if need be to protect us never ceases to amaze me. The military, in my opinion, is the best functioning government organization in the United States.

When at times I might get down because of our nation's direction, I think of the military and what those young men and women do each day and what hardships they endure. They are rewarded with very little and then often criticized, which irritates me. But thinking of them and what they accomplish is uplifting.

It is the call to action, the call to duty that in some respects is missing from the health care reform debate. What the politicians, business leaders and the American people must realize is that we have to come together and address the many failings of the current system, put aside partisan politics and treat this issue like a strategic military operation, in need of a reasonable course of action.

If this is to be the goal for health care moving forward, then we must step back and first assess what is wrong with the current system, otherwise we are building on a weak foundation that sits on sand. Again, as General Robert E. Lee said, it is our "duty" to finally get it right.

4

INVESTIGATING THE
INSURANCE INDUSTRY

Criticism may not be agreeable, but it is necessary.
It fulfills the same function as pain in the human body.
It calls attention to an unhealthy state of things.

– WINSTON CHURCHILL

WHILE THE UNITED STATES has the best health care system in place, it comes at a price that rises unnecessarily each year. This is due, in part, to the private sector's support of Medicare, Medicaid and the State Children's Health Insurance Plan (SCHIP).

What about those people with the ability to pay, but who opt out of acquiring insurance? These are not the "invincible" crowd alone. Approximately 70 percent of the uninsured cite high insurance premiums as the reason for opting out of coverage.

According to *At the Brink: Trends in America's Uninsured 1994-2007*, a report conducted by the State Health Access Data Assistance Center at the University of Minnesota, the average costs for an individual insurance policy have increased 61 percent—from $2,560 in 1996 to $4,118 in 2006. Nationwide, the amount that employees pay for an individual policy has increased by 79 percent, with wages in the U.S increasing only 10 percent over the same time period.

READ BETWEEN THE LINES

With five different 1,000-plus-page reform bills under consideration (which some politicians have admitted to not reading), it should again come as no surprise that misinformation has entered this critical debate. Regardless of which side of the aisle one falls, there is little gained from basing opinion merely on sound bites and posturing pundits.

A severe consequence of the sound-bite culture is that it's difficult to decipher what steps included in the bill will actually reform health care, so that boilerplate issues are addressed.

At a recent town hall meeting in Thousands Oaks, California, heated debates led to physical fights—one man's finger was bitten off. When people come to blows about health care and, as a result, need medical treatment, the situation is dire.

Among the issues currently, and historically, absent from the bill are federal regulation and the reform of the insurance industry. People without insurance impact our business model tremendously. Universal Health Services spends 11 to 12 percent of our revenue on bad debt, meaning we provide exceptional services for which we do not receive compensation.

Upwards of 60 percent of all insurance policies are employer provided. The average person doesn't understand the cost breakdown of what they are paying for as they do with their car insurance or homeowners insurance, for example. Across the 50 states, employees pay between 16 and 24 percent of the cost of their coverage.

According to the American Medical Association, only one in six employers providing insurance plans offer a choice of plans. Nationwide, the number of working uninsured adults has increased, with nearly one in five working adults in the uninsured column. The current administration, with a majority in Congress, has the ability to bring these issues to the bargaining table if it so chooses. For that matter, any administration in the last 30 plus years could have called for such regulation and avoided this aspect of our current situation.

What we have is a federal government that seems to protect the insurance companies, which focus their efforts on large business owners that can provide many policyholders. The small businessman—the tailor, or the auto body shop owner—is left out of the conversation. They have no leverage. And if an individual obtains a costly policy bought with after-tax dollars (approximately 20 percent higher than employer-provided insurance), he can only purchase policies in the state he resides. Is this fair?

A recent Commonwealth Fund report stated that between 1999 and 2008 employer-sponsored insurance premiums rose by 119 percent. If this growth rate is sustained, by 2020, they estimate it could rise by another 94 percent to an average of $23,842 per family. Included in the report was a state-by-state analysis. From 2003 to 2008, the average increase for family coverage was 33 percent. Indiana and North Carolina were the highest at 45 percent while Michigan, Texas and Ohio were the lowest with an increase of 25 percent. In 2008, the highest costs were reported in Indiana, Massachusetts, Minnesota and New Hampshire, where yearly family insurance premiums topped $13,500. The lowest states were Idaho, Iowa and Hawaii with average family premiums around $11,000.

In October 2009, the America's Health Insurance Plans commissioned an industry report prepared by PricewaterhouseCoopers that found that if the proposed health care legislation were passed, insurance rates would increase rather than decrease over time. According to the report, the increased premiums costs will likely cause people to wait until they are sick to obtain coverage. Other contributing factors include new taxes on health insurance plans, medical device makers and pharmaceutical manufacturers. The report found that the proposed reduction in Medicare spending would shift more costs to families. In addition, taxes on high-value plans are estimated to raise the cost of employer-provided coverage.

The system is broken. Sure, it is a cause for debate at town hall meetings and among pundits, but unless sound insurance regulation is entered into the bill, we will not achieve progressive health care reform but have more of the same: escalating premiums and more people entering the ranks of the uninsured in coming years.

HOW DO YOU KNOW WHEN IT GETS TOO HOT?

I've been happily married to my wife, Jill, for 41 years. We have three great kids: a son, Marc (who was recently named president of Universal Health Services, Inc.); two daughters, Marni and Abby; and a handful of high-energy grandchildren running around.

Jill grew up in the next borough over, in Queens. When we first met, she worked for the Department of Public Works. That was the mid-1960s. When the issue of our government running America's health care came to pass, Jill related stories to me from her days working for New York's bureaucracy. In her Manhattan office, they had a rule in the summer that when it reached 85 degrees, the office would be closed because there was no air-conditioning. Fine. If it was unreasonably hot, the workers couldn't work; fair enough. One person was placed in charge of gauging the temperature. Throughout the day people were consumed with how hot it was and continually checked with the man holding the thermometer. So maybe it hit the mark at 2:30 p.m. They anticipated when they could go home, not what they could accomplish before they went home. It upset Jill that her fellow employees weren't motivated but rather milled around waiting for five o'clock, or on hot days, for the sun to show its strength. This is not to say there weren't bright people working in her department; there were.

None of these people, however, were considered risk takers. They had the ability to accomplish more, but they had no incentive. Across the board, the idea was, as it is today, keep your nose clean, don't make any trouble, don't do too much work and you'll retire and get a pension. That is what it is all about. For some people this approach is fine, but when we consider similar government entities taking over a varied and complex system such as health care, it is no wonder people are rightfully concerned. Are you ready to let the government literally and figuratively check your temperature?

LOOK OVER YOUR SHOULDER

During the time period of the aforementioned anecdote, Medicare legislation was signed into law. For young people today, it's hard to understand that the going to the hospital in those days was a far different experience. A quick look back, however, gives a better understanding as to where we find ourselves today.

During the early 1950s, national health care expenditures represented 4.5 percent of the Gross National Product. While there was discussion of national health care reform, people focused on the Korean War to the detriment of the health care issue.

NATIONAL HEALTH CARE EXPENDITURES
1950s: 4.5% (Gross National Product)
2008: 17% (Gross Domestic Product)

NUMBER OF INSURANCE COMPANIES
1950s: Approximately 700
2008: Approximately 1,300

For the medical industry, it was a fertile period with new medications made available to treat a number of diseases, including glaucoma and arthritis. Additionally, new vaccines hit the market, preventing devastating childhood diseases such as polio.

Due to advancements, hospital costs nearly doubled in the 1960s. Doctors were focusing on specialty medicine with more frequency, and the federal government became concerned about a possible shortage of doctors across the board and pushed for expanded education in health-related fields.

Characteristics of Medicare's Beneficiaries

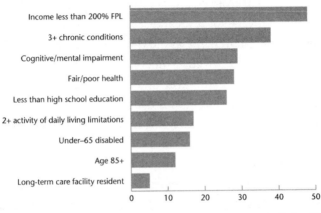

Source: Current Poplulation Survey; CMS Medicare Current Beneficiary Survey, 2006.

Approximately 700 insurance companies existed with 75 percent of Americans holding some form of private health insurance. As the new face of health care swept the nation, many of the elderly were left out of the equation, which in part gave rise to the Medicare platform.

When the Medicare bill was passed, serving approximately 18 million people, it wasn't looked upon as a program of huge expenditures, as it is today. The initial idea was for the government to assist an elderly person with a hospital bill they couldn't afford or a bill they needed assistance in paying.

Then, of course, came the unintended consequences. Doctors by nature are entrepreneurs. As more doctors became specialists, they called for more tests, including those patients receiving Medicare. This, in turn, spurred the insurance companies to offer more lines of insurance, and the industry expanded significantly.

So we went from essential care for the elderly to doctors ordering a myriad of tests and scans. Eventually, the whole program got out of hand, as did the insurance industry. That is the problem with government: a well-intentioned program gets bigger and bigger and more encompassing. Programs become broader and broader in coverage and before long, it breaks the bank. That is how these things work—all you need to do is study history.

In 1963, the Advisory Council on Social Security released a report that found that medical care costs for couples averaged about $442 yearly; costs for elderly couples with one or both members hospitalized averaged $1,220 yearly; for unmarried elderly people, average medical expenses for the year were $270.

Today, according to a recent study published by the American Hospital Association, the average cost for a hospital stay per day is $1,693, with South Dakota coming in on the low end at $869 and the District of Columbia at $2,381 per day. This is a great deal of money. Yes, inflation and technology have played a significant role in the increased prices, but so has an insurance industry that isn't given sufficient incentive to be more efficient.

APPLIED KNOWLEDGE

I have learned what doesn't work with bureaucratic government programs and done just the opposite in my company. Since the beginning, my idea was to keep the space in the office tight because if there is more space, then it will fill up. If people see space, they'll find a use for it. They find a need for an assistant or for more equipment, whatever the case might be.

If you build a huge corporate headquarters, it fills up. I've always taken a conservative, efficient approach. Nature abhors a vacuum, and people abhor empty space. We recently completed an extension to UHS's headquarters, which services 350 plus employees. It took 30 years before we did the project because we used up every inch of the existing facility before starting construction. We would find unused space and put off the project countless times until it became absolutely necessary.

Big government doesn't need to be this conservative, and that creates problems. The handwriting is on the wall.

CALL FOR REGULATION

I related the thermometer story because it underscores my stance on insurance reform. The latest survey from the Federal Agency for Healthcare Research and Quality stated that average American medical spending per person among 18- to 44-year-olds was $2,079 in 2006. Spending for 45- to 64-year-olds was $4,866, or a little more than double the younger demographic's figure.

INDIVIDUAL INSURANCE PLAN
COST SPIKES 61% IN 10 YEARS

1996: $2,560
2006: $4,118   ·

How do they come up with these figures? The answer is multifaceted. In our business model, for example, we are constantly negotiating with insurance companies. Essentially, we're trading off our services for their patient volume and reimbursement. It's a detailed and often lengthy process. We do the best we can at arm's length, and in turn, they do the best they can. Our goal is to get the highest reimbursement per day; theirs is to pay the least.

Insurance rates relate to how much an insurance company pays for hospital services and physicians, they then add on administrative costs and a profit margin. So, if they pay less, then theoretically, the premiums should be less. The more services we offer, the more attractive we are to the insurance company.

By and large, we negotiate market by market. Since each market in the nation is different, so are the terms. Our degree of interest in an insurance company varies, depending on how many lives/policies they have. They are interested in us, depending on what services we can provide. Perhaps most importantly, they are interested in our reputation. They are, in effect, selling our hospital to their clients once we have agreed on a contract.

Fortunately, I have never dealt personally with a situation where an insurance company denied coverage to my family members. I've read and, from business experience, understand that it happens. I find this infuriating and unfair. Federal and state regulations should be in place to take these companies to task for unfairly denying coverage. Are they currently in place? Not really.

The concept of attaining, or not attaining, insurance due

to "preexisting conditions" in certain circumstances may be unfair. Here is yet another example where reform is needed.

To draw an analogy, people have varying degrees of homeowners insurance. In recent years, our country has faced a slew of national disasters. Too many, it seems, insurance companies didn't deal with customers fairly when a legitimate claim was filed. The public opinion of insurance companies is often negative. When premiums are paid, everything is fine. When a claim is filed, it may be a different story. All too often, health insurance companies deserve the same perception.

Let's say a person has paid health insurance premiums for 10 years, and then the person changes jobs (and must reapply for employer-provided insurance). The insurance company reevaluates that person's health condition and ultimately denies coverage or places him or her in a different higher premium group because their health condition has degenerated or a new disease has surfaced. That's not fair.

We deal with insurance cases where a person is denied coverage, which means if we want to get paid, we must pursue the issue. We do this routinely because we have our own collection department well versed in handling claims; more times than not we know that the procedure should be covered.

There are situations where people are buying policies that are fraudulent. If a policy costs $12,000 for a family of four per year and someone finds a policy for $1,700 per year, a flag should be raised.

If someone is offered a bargain, there are likely exclusions in the fine print. Unfortunately, these polices are often directed at the lower income families trying to do the right thing, which is to have health insurance in place. They find out too late about the exclusions and are left without coverage, while the insurance company legally walks away due to the fine print. This is unfair.

In the end, you get what you pay for, and we need only look to the subprime mortgage mess that crippled the economy for proof. After the government pushed Freddie Mac and Fannie Mae into insolvency, the government moved into the mortgage business and what happened as a result? The answer, at the moment, is more trouble. Let's face it; the government doesn't manage many things well.

From my experience, more often that not, insurance companies that are refusing payment are usually playing the "stall" game. They will cite a missing image, file or signature in the submitted claim. Then there is a period of back and forth, and the insurance company hopes that we will not be able to produce requested materials and they can be relieved of payment on a technicality. At minimum, they have delayed the payment in an attempt to keep the money longer.

We, like all hospitals, have a department dedicated to insurance collections, so this becomes a nonsensical game that costs money and places patients in an unnecessary state of duress. And it's not just the private insurance companies that play this game. The federal government does, too.

If there were more transparency as a result of government reform, consumers would have more affordable insurance plans that clearly spell out what is covered and what is not covered. Consumers shop for auto insurance and can compare rates between Geico and Allstate, for example. Why aren't they afforded the same opportunity when it comes to health insurance?

SLIDING SCALE

For people that don't qualify for Medicare, Medicaid, SCHIP or other state-funded insurance plans, hospitals have to negotiate fees. A typical scenario is a person will come into one of our hospitals in need of services. They receive treatment, and he or she runs up a bill and may not have insurance. Often these are people who can afford insurance, but don't pay for coverage for various reasons, some of which were covered in previous chapters.

With these patients, we negotiate a payment plan. By and large, we don't always get 100 percent of our fees associated with the rendered services, but we manage to negotiate a fee that covers hospital expenses at the very least. It's a costly administrative process that increases the cost of doing business. We sit down with the individual and find out how much money they make and what they should be able to pay. We often offer him or her a discounted plan and provide a payment schedule. If these people were provided the opportunity to buy lower priced insurance, a tremendous amount of time and energy, collectively, would be saved.

There is a small part of our business, which is self-pay, that comprises approximately 10 percent of our total revenues. These people pay cash. No insurance coverage. We always offer patients a discount from paying the full charges.

A recent study supported by the Henry J. Kaiser Family Foundation found that uninsured patients are in some

ALAN B. MILLER

cases charged two and a half times more for hospital care than those covered by health insurance and more than three times the allowable amount paid by Medicare. As a result, the person who couldn't afford, or secure, health insurance due to cost, is then penalized when they do need care and are willing to pay for it. Why kick them when they are down?

INSURANCE RATIOS

Insurance companies haven't been on the sidelines when it comes to the issue of reform. Their industry is known for its ability to negotiate. America's Health Insurance Plans (ACHIP) told Congress during the summer of 2009 that they wanted the ability to charge seniors five times what they charge young people. This approach is not without logic as the 18 to 34 age demographic may spend $500 annually on health care where a senior (65 and older) spends eight to 10 times more each year.

The obvious issue is that a large majority of the younger demographic doesn't have health insurance, which raises the idea of instituting mandatory health insurance for all citizens over age 18. This controversial topic will be covered in subsequent chapters.

By and large, this younger demographic is healthy and doesn't need to go to the doctor regularly. However, this approach can create issues. Since this demographic, due to their relatively healthy nature, opt out of insurance, it removes the likelihood they will have yearly checkups. Unfortunately, a major problem could go undetected until it is too late. Then, when the problem is discovered, it negatively impacts the pricing system. For example, hospitals bills that are not paid are absorbed by the hospital, which in turn raises the price of procedures and tests for other patients.

The insurance ratio model segments demographics by age and likely liability and prices policies accordingly. This system is not without merit. Although AARP wants the ratio of two to one, the insurance industry is demanding a five to one ratio in order to play ball.

Insurance companies are quite astute at slicing ratios in different ways. For example, within the 18 to 34 demographic, they have subgroups (i.e. gender, etc.). They know by disease or procedure what they will have to expend, and actuaries adjust the policy accordingly.

By and large, the reason American businesses have been so successful throughout the years is that they have accurate information—we're information freaks. Actuaries are continually making adjustments with the intent of increasing return on their investment. It's the American way of doing business, plain and simple. By way of comparison, I sit on the Board of Directors of Penn Mutual Life Insurance Company, and the goal there is to get an 11 percent return on equity annually.

ASSESSING THE SITUATION

It is these nuanced issues, such as insurance ratios, surrounding the health care debate that gave rise to this book. I've written op-ed articles for *The Wall Street Journal,* appeared on CNBC and I've been interviewed on Fox News and the *Laura Ingraham Show*, among others. Aside from my public support of the malpractice reform in California in 1975, I haven't spoken out. However, issues such as insurance reform are too important to ignore, especially when there is so much at stake. The time is now.

We have a vehicle in need of repair. Malpractice and tort reform represent the failing engine, and the insurance industry is one of the tires losing air and is nearly flat. The American people are pumping unnecessarily overpriced fuel (in the form of rising insurance premiums) into the tank and getting horrible gas mileage.

We're nearly done assessing what's wrong with this vehicle we're calling health care reform, and soon we'll discuss ways to get her running in tip-top shape.

It's like Winston Churchill said, "Criticism may not be agreeable, but it is necessary."

5

INSURANCE AND HEALTH CARE

*Labor to keep alive in your breast that little
spark of celestial fire, called conscience.*

– GEORGE WASHINGTON

THE ISSUES SURROUNDING insurance coverage and reform are overarching. While the health care debate has in many respects raised more questions than answers for the American public, it has brought the insurance companies into the discussion, which is beneficial.

As previously discussed, the insurance industry is seeking to increase the number of those covered, specifically the 18 to 34 demographic, which would put them in the position to set ratios with regard to age and corresponding pricing guidelines.

Ostensibly, if the government were to mandate compulsory coverage within the private sector, then the insurance companies and hospitals would support reform because it would result in the following: More people paying premiums would benefit the insurance carriers. More patients getting treatment would benefit hospitals. Ultimately, Americans benefit because more people would gain access to health care.

The problem, or the trade-off, is that they can sell a policy, but they would have to cover all common lines of treatment from dental to acupuncture. This is a gray area and a cause for concern because it could change the stance of the various people coming to the bargaining table.

The insurance business model is straightforward—yes, it has loopholes and problems, but, theoretically, a company takes a large group of customers, aggregates pertinent information and then determines the appropriate premiums.

With a large enough pool, they have the money needed to pay a policyholder when a house burns down, and make a profit, too. However, if the insurance company only has eight policyholders and three houses are destroyed by fire, there is not enough insurance to cover the loss. This is one of the reasons companies selling health insurance are looking to expand the number of policyholders by bringing more people under the tent.

But a balance needs to be struck. As noted, there are problems with the insurance industry, which need to be addressed through regulation. At the same time, is it reasonable to demand they honor all preexisting medical conditions? If this is the case, then why would anyone need insurance when they are well?

Let's say an uninsured person goes to a doctor who delivers devastating news that he or she has cancer. The patient could then call an insurance company and ask for a policy. Does that sound fair? It's tantamount to someone who doesn't have any homeowner's insurance waking up to find his house burning. Can he call an insurance company explaining there is a fire in his basement, and ask for a policy immediately before the fire spreads to the roof?

Reasonable parameters must be established. If a person has worked for a company for a number of years and has paid into the system, then he or she shouldn't be denied coverage for any reason. On the other hand, a person shouldn't be able to call a company when they're in terrible shape—perhaps in need of a heart transplant—and expect full coverage. So, where is the middle ground?

On average, an insurance company keeps 15 to 25 percent of the premiums they collect. In 2007, Consumer Reports found that the nation's six biggest private health insurers collectively earned nearly $11 billion in profits in 2006. I support a fair profit margin as long as services are rendered.

To be clear, there are many upstanding insurance companies offering coverage. There are also exceptions that should be explored, specifically the cases where policyholders are underinsured or not aware of the limitations placed on their policies.

UNDERINSURANCE

Many Americans are underinsured and don't realize it until it is too late. Others do realize that they are underinsured and opt to purchase disaster insurance with deductibles upwards of $1,000. In some cases deductibles can be $5,000 to $10,000.

People make this decision for a variety of reasons, but for the most part, they are trying to lessen their monthly costs. The challenge is to reduce premiums for the employer, who can then pass the savings on to their employees, who will then have better coverage. This in turn would bring down our hospital costs.

THE UNDERINSURED

2003: 6 million

2007: 25 million

50% of underinsured opted against medical care.

Source: Commonwealth Fund.

While there is little data to support the levels of under-insurance nationwide, a 2008 survey by the Commonwealth Fund, a New York-based nonprofit that studies healthcare issues, found that roughly 25 million Americans are under-insured, an increase of 6 million from 2003. Commonwealth Fund defines "underinsured" as a person, or family, that pays more than 10 percent of their income on medical expenses.

Upwards of 50 percent of the underinsured opted against spending for medical care, including not seeing a doctor when sick, refusing recommended diagnostic tests and treatments and not filling prescriptions. The reason was associated with cost. Essentially, due to the current system, people are forced to gamble with their health.

As a result of not having adequate coverage, they may skip one too many appointments and miss a major health issue that, once diagnosed, may not be covered by their insurer. Insurance companies still make their profit, but hospitals, as covered in previous chapters, are left holding the bag and must absorb more bad debt.

A quick search for news articles on the topic of underinsured will yield many hard luck stories that underscore the problem. For example, a woman who lived in northern California operated a small winery business. She was bitten by a rattlesnake and required an overnight stay in the hospital, which included antivenom serum and morphine. The hospital bill was a purported $73,000, and her insurance company would only cover $3,000. She paid roughly $280 per month for her policy, which had a $500 deductible. She was under the impression that she had $50,000 in-hospital coverage. What she didn't realize was that there was a cap of $3,000 per day.

Eventually, the hospital reduced the bill to approximately $7,400 under a state program that limits charges for qualified low-income patients. This is an example of a flawed system.

ETHICAL OVERSIGHT

Reform and legislation to curb practices that leave Americans facing bankruptcy due to medical conditions and lack of insurance coverage should be a focal point of this health care debate.

Congress and other governmental bodies play an important role in legislating corporate governance standards and ethical behavior, but just because something is legal, doesn't mean it's ethical. The health care debate is a perfect example.

There have been cases reported where an insured person's policy is revoked after receiving a new diagnosis. According to the Department of Health and Human Services, certain insurance companies will examine the policyholder's initial questionnaire when there is a diagnosis of an expensive condition, such as cancer.

In most states, insurance companies can (legally) retroactively cancel an individual's policy if a condition were deemed not to be disclosed when the policy was issued. On the Department of Health and Human Services' website, it states that a policy would be canceled "...even if the medical condition is unrelated, and even if the person was not aware of the condition at the time." Additionally, "Coverage can also be revoked for all members of a family, even if only one family member failed to disclose a medical condition."

The House Committee on Energy and Commerce recently released a report that found that three large insurers rescinded roughly 20,000 policies in the course of five years, which saved the companies approximately $300 million in medical claims. Interestingly, the number of Medicare denials vastly exceeds the number of private insurance denials.

Of course, these statistics were released by the same administration that is behind health care reform. Again, consider the source; it can be a case of "liars figure and figures lie." On the other hand, we are presented with an opportunity for growth and compromise. Boiled down to the bare bones: if one party (Democrat) agreed to malpractice reform and the other party (Republican) pushed for insurance reform, for example, the monies saved would be tremendous and drastically change the focus of the debate because the figure "$1 trillion plus" would not have to enter into the picture.

So, can we fault the insurance industry for unethical practices? Sometimes, however, they are often operating legally as is the case with denying preexisting conditions. Again, we need to enact enforceable laws that will level the playing field. Insurance companies, like pharmaceutical companies, are entitled to make healthy profits, but only when they deliver on their promises.

CHARACTER BUILDING

When approaching an issue as encompassing as health care reform, it often helps to look back on our nation's history. At present, the country is divided on the issue. As a nation, we have a long history of division over major issues. In the end, we are all Americans and should be unified with the characteristics that built our country and afforded each of us the opportunity to overcome adversity.

Take George Washington, for example. If there is one word I would attach to him, especially during his early career, that word would be *perseverance*.

More than once the revolutionary army wanted to quit on Washington, and many in Congress were against him when things went badly. They didn't provide adequate payment or equipment to his men, who often didn't have blankets, shoes and ammunition. His accomplishments were unbelievable. Without him, we would not have the United States of America. He lost more battles than he won, but he never gave up on the war and the cause. Independence from England by defeating the redcoats was the goal, especially at a time when roughly half the country was still loyal to the British.

He had people angling for his job and generals working behind his back, imploring Congress to have him fired. His character was such that he persevered. In some respects, it seemed like a miracle that this man was in the field for eight years undeterred, surmounting obstacle after obstacle. It was as a result of surrounding himself with enough capable people—men of character—like himself, that he was able to prevail in the end.

We can look to our forefathers to realize that standing on principle is often a hard thing to do. Now, our current health care reform is hardly equivalent to Washington's plight, but there are lessons to be learned.

I believe that, for the most part, the people on either side of this debate want what in the end is best for the American public. Does self-interest exist? Of course. However, it has been my experience that selfish approaches collapse under their own weight in the final analysis.

The lack of agreement between the two camps isn't about providing quality health care to America. It is the question of how we get there without bankrupting the nation. Less government and more competition within the segments that make up the entire system should be the goal. People shouldn't stick so strongly to party lines on this issue because in the end, it comes down to identifying the most appropriate, sustainable health care reform model. The government can print money, fill up space and make promises, but even a regulated private sector only succeeds when there is a sound business model in place. All others fail and are forgotten.

Every government official and private sector representative coming to the table for this debate should keep in mind a message George Washington sent on September 14, 1775, to the ambitious Benedict Arnold, who was always seeking higher office: "Every post is honorable in which a man can serve his country."

MONOPOLY

I firmly believe that competition makes for better products, lower prices and, in the case of health care, better coverage. This is true in the insurance industry, however, in many states there are only a few competing insurance companies.

While nationwide there are approximately 1,300 insurance companies, state regulations are such that competition is often removed from the equation. In some states, for example, the only game in town is BlueCross BlueShield, considered by most to provide satisfactory coverage and reasonable rates. In a state like Alabama, for instance, they have approximately 80 to 90 percent of the market share. Other states may have more than one or two insurers, perhaps up to 10, but there is usually a dominant company. Despite its good reputation, why shouldn't other providers be allowed to compete against BlueCross BlueShield?

Insurance Monopoly in Alabama

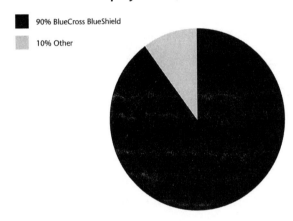

■ 90% BlueCross BlueShield

10% Other

According to studies conducted by Health Care for America NOW! (HCAN!) and the American Hospital Association (AHA), Anthem BlueCross BlueShield, Inc. has 78 percent of the market in Maine. In Idaho, BlueCross of Idaho and Regence BlueShield of Idaho together total 75 percent of the state's insurance market. These figures do not include Medicare, Medicaid or State Children's Health Insurance Program enrollment.

States Dominated by Two Health Plans with More Than 50% of Total Insured
(By Market Share)

Census estimates, served by the listed companies.

State	Market Leader	Market Share as % of Population	Combined Market Share
Minnesota	Blue Cross and Blue Shield of Minnesota	47.79%	76.20%
	Medica Health Plans	28.41%	
Delaware	Blue Cross Blue Shield of Delaware	59.33%	75.89%
	Coventry Health and Life Insurance Company	16.56%	
Hawaii	Hawaii Medical Service Association	54.40%	71.72%
	Kaiser Permanente	17.32%	
North Dakota	Blue Cross Blue Shield of North Dakota	62.53%	67.88%
	Humana Inc.	5.35%	
Alabama	Blue Cross and Blue Shield of Alabama	64.22%	66.31%
	Humana Inc.	2.09%	
Illinois	Blue Cross and Blue Shield of Illinois	57.22%	61.42%
	Aetna Inc.	4.20%	

State	Market Leader	Market Share as % of Population	Combined Market Share
Massachusetts	Blue Cross Blue Shield of Massachusetts	46.71%	60.36%
	Harvard Pilgrim Health Plan	13.65%	
Michigan	Blue Cross Blue Shield of Michigan	49.76%	54.99%
	Health Alliance Plan of Michigan	5.23%	
New Jersey	Horizon Blue Cross Blue Shield	36.26%	52.41%
	Aetna Inc.	16.15%	
South Dakota	Wellmark Blue Cross and Blue Shield of South	39.81%	52.31%
	DAKOTA	12.50%	
Iowa	Wellmark Blue Cross and Blue Shield of Iowa	47.80%	51.45%
	Humana, Inc.	3.65%	

SOURCE: Compiled by Atlantic Information Services, Inc. editors from AIS's Directory of Health Plans: 2009 and insurance department filings.

The first question that should come to mind is: where is the regulation? This is not a new issue for American business; it was tackled on July 2, 1890, when the Sherman Antitrust Act was signed into law. As a refresher, the bill requires the United States Federal Government to investigate and pursue trusts, companies and organizations suspected of violating the act. It was a groundbreaking federal statute, the first of its kind to curb cartels and monopolies.

When you don't have monopolies, everyone benefits, except the monopolist. Has the Sherman Antitrust Act been discussed during the debate?

In 1945, the insurance industry took a huge leap toward the quasi-insurance monopolies we experience today when the Supreme Court ruled on the United States versus South-Eastern Underwriters Association.

The case came to the Supreme Court in 1944 on appeal from a northern Georgia district court. At the time, the South-Eastern Underwriters Association maintained 90 percent of the market for commercial and residential fire insurance and other insurance lines in six neighboring southern states. They established rates at noncompetitive levels and used intimidation tactics, including boycotts, to thwart competition.

The court ruled that insurance could be regulated by the federal government, or, in short, insurance fell under interstate commerce. This is known as the McCarran-Ferguson Act, which doesn't regulate insurance, nor mandate that states regulate insurance. What it does do is allow Congress to pass laws that impact the regulating of the insurance industry.

The real catch is that the act provides that federal antitrust laws cannot apply to the "business of insurance" as long as the state regulates that area. The federal antitrust laws only apply in cases citing boycott, coercion and intimidation.

Before the decision was rendered by the court, it was

the then-conventional wisdom that insurance did fall under interstate commerce and, therefore, could be regulated by the Commerce Clause and the Sherman Antitrust Act. The Supreme Court ruling included the following explanation:

> "Any enactment by Congress either of partial or of comprehensive regulations of the insurance business would come to us with the most forceful presumption of constitutional validity. The fiction that insurance is not commerce could not be sustained against such a presumption, for resort to the facts would support the presumption in favor of the congressional action. The faction therefore must yield to congressional action and continues only at the sufferance of Congress.
>
> Congress also may, without exerting its full regulatory powers over the subject, and without challenging the basis or supplanting the details of state regulation, enact prohibitions of any acts in pursuit of the insurance business which substantially affect or unduly burden or restrain interstate commerce."

When we flash forward to today's market, the McCarran-Ferguson Act legally allows states to regulate business and insurance. The states and the legislators have a vested interest in getting money from lobbyists who have an interest in talking about insurance and related services.

Next thing you know, mandates are discussed. Every segment of the health care industry providing forms of insurance, like dental, psychiatric, chiropractic, yoga, massage and the lists goes on, seeks to be included in mandated coverage.

On the other side of the coin, there are jobs to consider. Each state has an insurance commissioner who oversees a department. There are investigators and regulators. A whole state-based industry is required. The state creates another big bureaucracy with big budgets to oversee and administer. The insurance companies again are operating "legally," and in turn politicians and departments continue to operate this somewhat oversized system. Who ultimately suffers? Policyholders do. If the federal government got its act together, they could reduce the size of these state departments.

If federal insurance regulation were introduced, would some people lose their jobs on a state level? Yes. However, this is not a partisan issue; this would impact both sides of the aisle. It's a catch-22. Does a small minority of government workers get to keep their jobs so that an often-protected insurance industry can continue to operate with limited competition? These are times when tough decisions need to be made.

After the fall of Fort Washington in 1776, General George Washington wrote, "If I were to put a curse on my worst enemy, it would to be to wish him in my position now. I just do not know what to do. It seems impossible to continue my command in this situation, but if I withdraw, all will be lost."

In the face of defeat and self-doubt, Washington stuck to his guns for the betterment of the country—not simply for himself or his command. We, as a nation, are facing an uncertain future; we should heed Washington's words and not give up or give in to a health care reform bill that doesn't achieve the necessary goals.

SINGLE PAYER IS NO PUBLIC OPTION

*Money is power, and in that government which pays
all the public officers of the states will all political
power be substantially concentrated.*

– ANDREW JACKSON

THE MAJOR ISSUES SURROUNDING the health care reform debate have been presented and discussed. Now we can focus on solutions, beginning by addressing the issue of a single-payer health care system.

So we're clear, the single-payer model is a government-managed health care system where all payments to doctors, hospitals and health care providers come from a single source. In short, there is no middleman. The single-payer system is the United Kingdom's socialized medicine. The public option in the United States would likely lead to single payer or universal health care; it's ultimately socialized medicine.

When all these different terms are used, it's no wonder the average person is confused by this debate. Ultimately, there is no option in the public option. As a result of heated debates, the American public is beginning to realize what this means. The government is not going to compete with insurers; they are going to drive them out of business. Advocates of the single-payer platform say that hospitals, for example, would survive implementation of the single-payer system if they learned to operate more efficiently.

For the balance of my career, I've continually sought new ways to become more efficient. If I didn't, my company would not have lasted for 30 years and be as successful as it is today. The economic conditions of the past few years have forced most businesses to reduce expenses and increase efficiency. So, this counterpoint doesn't hold water with me. Additionally, Americans have come to expect the best health care in the world, and in order to provide that care, hospitals must continue to invest in advanced medical technology, salaries for well-trained nurses and technicians, and state-of-the-art facilities.

If hospitals were required to operate solely on the revenue from a single-payer system, they could no longer afford to provide the care that Americans rightly deserve. Medicare already operates below cost, and if the program was offered to all, it would have dire consequences. For those who question this opinion, my company's experience with healthcare in the United Kingdom further illustrates my position.

ACROSS THE POND

In 1985, Universal Health Services made a major strategic decision to invest in the U.K. by building two private hospitals and acquiring a third. At the time, Great Britain was devoting less of its Gross National Product to health care than any other industrialized nation. As a consequence, the National Health Service, the U.K.'s publicly funded *health service*, was underfunded and wasn't able to keep pace with new technologies or the building of new hospitals. This presented a unique opportunity.

One of our hospitals, the newly built London Independent with 102 beds, was in the neighborhood of the London Hospital, which had approximately 1,000 beds. It had been operating for nearly 100 years. I recall there was a plaque on a wall of the operating suite dating back to the 1880s. Upon touring the facility, what I found most disconcerting was the spiral staircase, six stories high in the center of the hospital. It was enclosed with wire mesh. Essentially it was a firetrap—a fire funnel. The antiquated state of the building was astounding. There didn't seem to be building codes in place. And if there were, they weren't enforced, placing patients in potential danger.

During this time period, approximately 900,000 people were on National Health Services' waiting lists for various procedures. There were, however, those who needed and could afford private health care insurance. This gave rise to our business.

We will not operate a hospital that is ill-equipped. To this end, we invested in our hospital and attracted leading doctors. With leading doctors in place, great nurses and practitioners followed. Our reputation spread, and in two years, our patient volume increased by 40 percent.

As a result of our innovation and success, the London Hospital often came to us to borrow equipment. They couldn't compete with us, nor could they keep up with their demand. It was their patients who literally suffered—caught in a failing system.

Doctors would test for cancer, for example, and not be able to provide results for three to four weeks. It was inhuman. When I learned that our administration was lending out equipment, I was surprised. The doctors would explain that their associates, doctors down the street, were without resources. I inquired why these patients couldn't be sent directly to our hospital, and the response was simply that these people did not have coverage.

We were placed in an awkward position, and in the end, we lent out our equipment for operations like a craniotomy. On one hand, it was the right thing to do, but on the other, we were better equipped than the government to administer health care. We were in effect subsidizing them, on top of the taxes we paid.

At the time, in addition to the single-payer system, there was a private insurance segment of five million people. Citizens paid their taxes, which were very high, and if they wanted to get treated without waiting on line, they purchased private insurance as well. These people ended up paying twice. That's hardly efficient.

This was my first opportunity to see the U.K.'s poorly constructed socialized health care system. The experience convinced me that under a single-payer system, with tight budgets and rationing, hospitals do not receive the money required to provide top quality care.

While the Thatcher government tried to promote increased privatization of the country's health care system, it didn't work mainly because the nation has a class system. It's interesting because the average, class-conscious Briton seems to resent people with money. The nurses and technicians who worked in government hospitals also resented patients that could afford "pay beds," a section for those with insurance, who avoided the waiting line.

One year before an election, the National Health Services

would have what I called a "field-clearing" initiative. Officials would contact us and ask if we could do a certain number of operations, let's say 5,000 hernia operations, because the waiting period was so long. While British people are stoic by and large, many are forced to suffer for anywhere from weeks to 18 or 24 months for an operation. For those who can't afford additional private insurance, this remains the reality.

The government found the money and, in an attempt to assuage the people at election time, would pay companies like mine to cover their weakness. It was pathetic. Is this what the American people want?

Single-payer systems have proven to be inadequate in countries such as the United Kingdom. After eight years, we exited that market. Recent news stories out of the United Kingdom report that women, on occasion, are giving birth in hospital elevators, parking garages, bathrooms and midwives' offices. While these reports might be the exception rather than the rule, the U.K.'s single-payer system seemingly has gotten worse rather than better over the years.

In June 2009, the NHS released a report which found that 236,316 patients were forced to wait more than 18 weeks between general practitioner referral and admission to the hospital for treatment.

Salaries for bureaucrats in the U.K. system have risen considerably even as inadequate health practices continue. According to a recent study published in the *Daily Mail*, in 2007 and 2008, nearly £1.2 billion was spent on administrators and clerical staff in Primary Care Trusts, a government provider of primary and community services. This marked an increase of 81 percent since 2003. To illustrate how wasteful this bureaucratic system is, the NHS spent less than half the aforementioned amount on anti-cancer drugs in 2008, which meant certain patients were denied life-prolonging medication.

DEATH PANELS?

The majority of people in America are satisfied with the care they receive. So, it is important that we judiciously change only the areas in need of improvement.

Take, for example, Medicare reimbursements to hospitals that fail to cover the actual cost of providing services. The Medicare Payment Advisory Commission (MedPAC), an independent congressional advisory agency, says hospitals received 94.1 cents for every dollar they spent treating Medicare patients in 2007. MedPAC projects that number to decline to 93.1 cents for every dollar spent in 2009, for an operating shortfall of 7 percent. An AMA study reported 2,840 of the nation's hospitals lost money serving Medicare patients.

Medicare underfunds because hospitals subsidize the care they provide with revenue received from patients who have commercial insurance. Without that revenue, hospitals couldn't afford to treat those covered by Medicare. In effect, everyone with insurance is subsidizing the Medicare shortfall, which grows larger each year. When politicians propose Medicare for all, they don't realize that the program underpays providers.

Presently, MedPAC has 17 commissioners who are appointed by the comptroller general for a three-year term. In addition to advising Congress on payments to private health care plans participating in Medicare and to providers in Medicare's traditional fee-for-service program, MedPAC also analyzes access to care, quality of care, and other issues affecting Medicare.

When the issue of "death panels," an unfortunately blunt term, is brought up, we have to remember that government involvement in certain aspects of end-of-life decisions is already in place. In 1992, under a mandate put forth by President George H.W. Bush, the government required hospitals to ask adult patients if they had a living will, or "advance directive." If the patient was without one, and wanted one, the hospital was required to provide assistance. So, the idea of the government getting involved with certain aspects of end-of-life decisions already exists.

The difference now is the House bill permits Medicare to pay doctors for voluntary counseling sessions that address end-of-life issues. Doctor-patient conversations could include making a close relative or a trusted friend a health care proxy, discussing hospice as an option for the terminally ill, as well as giving information on available medications for people suffering from chronic discomfort or pain.

Another bill brought forward earlier this summer would significantly empower MedPAC, which would limit Congress's involvement in Medicare payment policy. The current MedPAC would give way to a federal "infrastructure for delivery system reform." If the bill were passed as part of health reform legislation, the members of the House of Representatives and the Senate would need a majority vote to override MedPAC. In effect, legislators would be largely unable to monitor MedPAC's payment decisions.

The Federal Reserve's Board of Governors would be the

model for the new MedPAC Commission with regard to the appointment process and policy oversight. The Medicare program still would be managed by the Centers for Medicare and Medicaid Services (CMS).

Presidential power also would increase dramatically because the president, with the advice and consent of Congress, would be responsible for appointing full-time members to MedPAC's board (11 people in total). The two non-voting members would be the Secretary of Health and Human Services (HHS) and the CMS Administrator.

As noted, I have operated hospitals in the United Kingdom, as well as France, which also has socialized medicine, and witnessed firsthand the central control of health care. In the U.K., the central control is under the National Institute for Health and Clinical Excellence (NICE), an organization that controls the health care of approximately 60 million Brits.

Both the U.K. and France try to ration health care on a reasonable basis. Who makes the decision as to who gets what? A group of appointed experts makes that determination. This sounds similar to the proposed MedPAC overhaul, doesn't it?

If health care becomes rationed, the nation's elderly population will certainly be the hardest hit demographic. In the U.K., NICE has the ability to accept or reject drugs and procedures. It is not surprising that with this approach they are ranked 15th out of 22 European Union countries in cancer survival rates.

America, however, leads the word in advanced pharmaceuticals and survival rates across many medicals fronts. When we look at states like Tennessee and Massachusetts, which have implemented some form of public option, we see certain disaster. Yes, the uninsured rates drops, but at what cost? Taxes are on the rise, people are waiting longer for health care and the bureaucracy becomes larger and larger.

We needn't look far for answers. While a public option or socialized medicine is presented as an attractive alternative, the problem is who pays in the end? Payment unfortunately comes in two forms: higher taxes and inadequate health care.

EXAMPLES ON THE HOME FRONT

During a recent interview, I was asked what impact Senator Ted Kennedy's passing would have on the current debate. As most people know, government-run, socialized medicine was an initiative he fought hard for during his entire tenure as the senior senator from Massachusetts. Of course, it is unfortunate that he passed, as he was considered to be a great senator. And while his political career will forever be tied to this issue for some, his death will not likely have a lasting impact on the outcome of the debate.

Among the states that have implemented some type of government-controlled health care services are Maine, Massachusetts, Tennessee and Hawaii.

Let's take a look at "the lion" of the Senate's Massachusetts, as it has been cited for comparison to a proposed national model. The state implemented a universal coverage program in 2006, driven and touted by the former governor of Massachusetts and Republican Mitt Romney. This was prior to his run for the Republican presidential nomination. He may have thought he would ride it into the White House. It seems the poor house is a more likely destination.

Initially, it was an insurance exchange program where private insurers would have the opportunity to compete. Shortly after launching the program, however, it was comprised of government mandates, fines, increased taxes and lawsuits.

To date, the costs are escalating far beyond what was estimated. This should not come as a surprise. The cost was supposed to be $1.04 billion in 2006, and in the fiscal period ending 2010, it is forecasted to be $1.75 billion, or higher. That represents an error of 75 percent.

What has been the result? The waiting list to see an internist has gone from 33 days in 2006-2007, to 53 days in 2009. Only 52 percent of internists will accept a new patient. Coverage costs have risen.

From inception to June 2008, the uninsured dropped from 8.3 percent to an estimated 2.6 percent, which is the positive in this dark cloud—the "no-cost public option." Before implementation, the number of uninsured was estimated at 630,000. Today, approximately 432,000 residents have been removed from that list.

THE MASSACHUSETTS HEALTH CARE REFORM MODEL

2006 Estimated Cost: $1.04 billion in 2006
2010 Estimated Cost: $1.75 billion
2006 Estimated Wait to See Internist: 33 days
2009 Estimated Wait to See Internist: 53 days

A facetious joke going around Massachusetts is, "Free insurance is getting very expensive." If this same model were implemented on a national level, a platform commonly called Obamacare, the estimated cost would be in the neighborhood of $1 trillion. If we are use Massachusetts as the model, the country could see the costs jump to $1.75 trillion, or more. Is this a reasonable thing to do?

As discussed earlier, state-regulated insurance gave way to bureaucracy and well-paid lobbyists. In just three short years, Massachusetts health care lobbyists have successfully added 16 types of coverage that now fall under the mandate. These include items such as hormone replacement therapy, non-invitro fertility services, orthotics, lay midwives and pediatric specialists. While some of these items are important, the list is expected to grow with the Massachusetts Legislature currently considering more than 70 additional requirements. As a result, premiums will have to dramatically rise. So in the end, what was accomplished?

DOCTORS IN DEMAND

While the number of uninsured has been estimated at nearly 48 million, my estimate, as previously noted, is far lower. The American Academy of Family Physicians recently released a report that found that 40,000 primary care physicians will be required within the next decade to handle the influx of patients, nationally. My figure of uninsured is approximately 16 million, or roughly 25 percent of the generally accepted number, will still require 10,000 new primary care physicians within in the next 10 years.

Soaring malpractice insurance rates and the unfortunate need to practice defensive medicine has deterred many would-be doctors from the profession, especially in the field of primary care. The Association of American Medical Colleges recently reported that the rate of first-year enrollees in U.S. medical schools has declined steadily since 1980. If this pattern continues, the United States will have approximately 159,000 fewer doctors than it needs by 2025.

And while supporters of the health care reform bill claim that more people will be able to afford quality health care, many doctors have raised eyebrows over the proposed legislation. In late September 2009, *Investor's Business Daily* and TechnoMetrica released a IBD/TIPP poll that found a staggering 72 percent of doctors disagreed with the administration's claim that the government can cover "47 million" more people with quality care at lower costs. For the poll, 1,376 practicing physicians were polled randomly, over a period of two weeks.

The American Medical Association (AMA), which has supported elements of the proposed reform bills, doesn't support a public option (they contend it would lower doctor fees). The AMA represents approximately 20 percent of the physicians practicing in the United States.

If Congress passed the health care reform bill, four out of nine doctors (45 percent) polled said they would consider leaving their practice or take an early retirement. In 2006, the government estimated that there were roughly 800,000 doctors practicing in the nation. If we extrapolate the aforementioned poll data, 360,000 doctors would seriously consider leaving the profession.

Today, the doctor to patient ratio is 2.4 to 1,000 and is

below the average 3.1 for members of the Organization for Economic Cooperation and Development, which compares policies of the leading nations.

A 2009 Physician Workforce Study found that the primary care specialties of family medicine and internal medicine are in short supply for a fourth straight year. The percentage of primary care practices closed to new patients is the highest ever recorded.

Along with family and internal medicine, seven of 18 specialties—dermatology, neurology, urology and vascular surgery—are in short supply. The survey found that recruitment and retention of physicians is an escalating problem, particularly at community hospitals and with primary care. Without doctors, we have no medical model. These are scary numbers.

COST OF DOING BUSINESS

Alex Rodriguez of the New York Yankees earns $28 million per year. Many business owners make close to $5 million per year. Does every baseball player and businessperson make this amount of money? No, only the best performers.

What this does demonstrate though is that a person at the top of his field in the United States can do very well. A motivated person stands to make a significant living and that is an incentive for everyone.

However, when you come back to this misguided philosophy, call it socialism or whatever you like, which basically says that making a great deal of money is obscene, we run into a basic misunderstanding. The people who hold this view don't seem to understand that incentives and rewards are the basis of our capitalistic system. The alternative is a bureaucracy charged with redistributing wealth, which is a frustrating place to be. Consider your last trip to the Department of Motor Vehicles, for example, then multiply that by an exponential factor and you begin to see a picture of government-run health care.

By way of comparison, take a look at Russia or Cuba—study all the failed states that have tried systems other than capitalism, such as communism and socialism. I understand that in the 1920s and 1930s, communism by and large was attractive because supposedly it would take care of everybody. What it did was eliminate incentive and efficiency. Where did these states wind up? Their production dropped and innovation disappeared. The people on top lived a life of luxury. The average people suffered. Now, it has been well recognized as a failed system.

My company and others in the private hospital sector are doing the government a service because we are investing heavily in facilities and technologies. We provide services similar to nonprofits and we pay taxes as well. We have to generate a return on our equity, we have to attract capital, we have to invest the capital and we have to pay the same wages and expenses as nonprofits. For example, their nurses and our nurses receive the same compensation. On top of this, we pay nearly 40 percent in taxes. How, and why, can we do it? Answer: not-for-profit organizations, as a result of lacking incentive, are inefficient and their shortcoming has allowed for the creation of a viable private market.

My company is not bureaucratic or overstaffed. Our business model is based on incentive and motivation, which allows us to perform efficiently. We are high-quality operators, and it is our practice to attract high-quality medical staff. Superior doctors will not put up with equipment that is not first rate. Since we own and operate the hospitals, we are responsible. My question is: would the federal government be able to compete, and expend, at this level? The United Kingdom's National Health Service couldn't keep up.

A single piece of equipment can cost $2 million. For example, a da Vinci Surgical System costs approximately $1.5 million. This advanced apparatus allows doctors to perform complex, minimally invasive surgeries using robotic manipulators. Staying competitive includes providing our doctors, nurses and technicians with the leading tools of the trade. The fixed cost in a hospital is enormously expensive. Every year we purchase numerous pieces of costly equipment. Technology becomes obsolete quickly.

There is one example after another of the benefits of advanced technologies, but again these are high cost items that have to be paid for whether we have 10 patients or 1,000. If payments aren't made by patients and insurance companies because of defaults or the like, the hospital is left with the bill.

LESSONS FROM KATRINA

We operated four acute care hospitals in and around New Orleans: Methodist Hospital, Lakeland Medical Pavilion, Chalmette Medical Center and Virtue Street Pavilion. When Katrina hit, we lost all these operations. The areas where these hospitals were located were considered poor.

Many of our patients were taken from us by the federal government to a centralized point, and we weren't exactly sure where these patients were headed. We set up a phone bank in our office to assist in locating patients and advising their families.

We were extremely frustrated because we were fielding calls from concerned family members asking where their mother or brother was. We didn't have a definitive answer because we were instructed by the government officials to take certain patients to airports for relocation but were not given information as to their final destinations.

It became our job to find the patients that the government displaced. Our phone banks were staffed 24 hours a day. To assist in the efforts on the ground, we contracted for planes and helicopters, private contractors to bring water, fuel for generators, supplies including food and various pieces of medical equipment to our hospitals. The government controlled the air space. At the airport, they established a command center.

The Federal Emergency Management Agency (FEMA) confiscated our supplies using the word "commandeer" as an explanation for taking our goods and services. Their operation was disorganized. Since we were the hospitals, to whom was the government going to give our supplies? What's more important in this type of situation, than a hospital willing to go the extra mile? When the U.S. Army came on the scene, a sense of order was established. Until that point, our good efforts were actually thwarted by the federal government. This is yet another example of an inefficient government operation.

VETERANS ADMINISTRATION HOSPITAL

The Veterans Health Administration operates approximately

150 hospitals. Many of the doctors practicing at our hospitals will volunteer their time and services at various locations around the country. The health care is variable depending on location, the equipment is usually dated and in need of upgrading.

This is not to say there aren't beneficial aspects to the VA model. It is a military operation that gives the organization a better foundation than other government-operated health care operations. Across the board, however, it is considered a troubled system. If you talk to most veterans, they would likely tell you that they wouldn't go to the VA hospital if they had the option of going to a private hospital.

Walter Reed Army Medical Center received a lot of negative press in recent years for the state of its operations. If you think about it, throughout the years, President Eisenhower, and other famous veterans, went there for care. Since the hospital is located in Washington, D.C. and receives high-profile patients, I would be surprised if this location is not the best of the best, which seemingly isn't saying much for other VA hospitals located around the country. All Americans deserve affordable health care, but it is shameful if our veterans are not rewarded with excellent care for their sacrifices.

PHYSICIAN PRACTICE MANAGEMENT COMPANIES

When we begin to investigate aspects of government-run health care, we fortunately have history on our side. As the saying goes, "Those who don't study history are doomed to repeat it."

Not long ago, physician practice management companies were touted as the next big venture in providing health care for Americans. Companies were created to buy practices from doctors, with the thought that aggregating size and support would bring efficiencies.

When the companies bought these practices, and the older doctors cashed out, the younger doctors, nurses and technicians had their salaries reduced to support the purchase price. What happened is the younger professionals basically got the short end of the stick.

A young guy—maybe 34, just out of medical school, highly educated and motivated, carrying $150,000 in debt instead of leaving the starting gate at $125,000 per year, is offered a job at $95,000. This lowering of salaries resulted from the amount of money that was spent on acquiring medical practices.

The concept ultimately failed. The leading reason was that a company tried to manage and regulate a profession that historically wasn't manageable. In fact, and as I said before, doctors are among the country's traditional entrepreneurs. This is the beauty of American medicine: hard-working, bright doctors providing excellent care to their patients.

While some specialty physician practice management companies managed to succeed, the percentage was low and the movement by and large was a failure. The only winners were the older doctors who sold their practices but stayed on in a limited capacity. They played golf on Wednesdays and Fridays, saw few patients and punched out at four o'clock—good for them I suppose, but it wasn't good for patients. That's the lesson. When a company or private sector movement takes a chance and fails, it goes away. When the government fails, the amount invested usually doubles. It's not the government's money, it's yours and mine.

FOCUS ON THE GOOD

I don't believe in hiring people who are not motivated. Doctors are willing to stay late and work long hours to make a certain income, which is usually on the high end. They value their independence. They're willing to work and provide health care as long as they have the ability to increase their earnings. I admire this approach. They have traditionally fought socialized medicine at every turn for this reason. If their respective ability to succeed in this entrepreneurial fashion is hampered, it would be a great shame.

There is, however, a segment of the medical profession, including doctors, who focus on lifestyle more than entrepreneurship. These doctors are happy to work a nine to five shift—often they are emergency medicine doctors who don't have the 24-hour stress of a patient load. They don't want late-night calls or to be bothered while on vacation. They are willing to trade the upside (lifestyle) for the convenience of not operating a practice. I'm not saying these are not terrific, well-meaning doctors, but their hours are limited.

My support of independent doctors is solid, but that is not to say they are not difficult to deal with at times—whether it is a request for the latest equipment or whatever the case may be. I encourage this approach because it means they are looking to provide exceptional care and will not be satisfied with anything less. While now I don't deal directly with doctors as much as I used to, I'm always happy to talk to a doctor if the conversation is based on what is good for their patients.

When a doctor is supported in this manner—putting the patient's comfort and concerns first—then the patient believes in the doctor and sees him or her as an advocate. As a result, he wants to maintain relations with that doctor. If that relationship is threatened for any reason, he gets understandably upset. The government should not seek to put bureaucrats between a doctor and his or her patient, or ration the care they can prescribe.

When I hear some imply that doctors do unnecessary procedures to make extra money, it misses the heart of the issue entirely. It's denigrating. Doctors go into this business for the love of medicine and helping people. It's obscene to think otherwise. I relate to my employees often that I believe people who are drawn to health care sincerely want to help people. Sure they want to make a good living, but they are drawn to the industry for the most admirable of reasons.

After leaving Wharton, my first career was in advertising working at Young & Rubicam in New York. I learned valuable lessons about entrepreneurship and risk-taking. At the time, I could barely scramble an egg but was instrumental in developing Graham Kerr into a nationally recognized chef by making *The Galloping Gourmet* with Graham Kerr a nationally syndicated television program. In the beginning, I carried two audition tapes trying to place the show on TV stations. One audition tape was Kerr cooking Chicken Polese. I was dating Jill at the time and made her the dish because I had watched it so many times that I could do it blindfolded. Luckily, it turned out to be her favorite.

In 1969, a friend called from Wharton with an idea for a new business. My entrepreneurial spirit took hold, and I left the advertising world to join American Medicorp, a start-up hospital company. After a few years, we hit financial troubles and the chairman left the company. These were difficult, trying times. I became CEO and managed to right the ship, and turn the company profitable which attracted a hostile takeover by Humana in 1978. This was devastating to me and the other senior management.

At the time I was faced with the decision whether to return to the advertising world where I had done very well, or stay in health care. After a period of introspection, I found more meaning in the health care field. The advertising industry is extremely important to the success of the country; I did it for eight years. But I was faced with a choice, and I simply felt better about a career in health care. I decided to put my energy and talents into a new venture: Universal Health Services.

As the health care debate unfolds and the ramifications of a single-payer system are realized, I feel it is important to recognize the entrepreneurial spirit of doctors and other health care professionals who want to maintain control of their respective careers.

The wisdom Andrew Jackson's imparted so many years ago applies to our current debate on health care. We must be careful where "political power in concentrated."

$$\boxed{7}$$

RECOMMENDATIONS ON
TORT REFORM

Nobody can acquire honor by doing what is wrong.
– THOMAS JEFFERSON

I CAN BARELY CONTAIN MYSELF when it comes to the issue of tort reform of medical malpractice. Without much needed reforms to limit jury awards for noneconomic damages, the cost of malpractice insurance will continue to rise. That, in turn, will increase the exodus of physicians from the particularly vulnerable specialties such as obstetrics, orthopedics and neurosurgery.

What is the result of rampant, uncontrolled malpractice lawsuits? It becomes increasingly difficult for Americans to secure treatment, and it's more expensive when they can. The fact that tort reform is barely mentioned in any of the proposed bills boggles the mind.

DIVIDED WE STAND

During the aforementioned speech on health care reform to the joint session of Congress on September 9, 2009, President Barack Obama said that Republicans have "long insisted that reforming our medical malpractice laws can help bring down the cost of health care." He then continued, "I don't believe malpractice reform is a silver bullet, but I have talked to enough doctors to know that defensive medicine may be contributing to unnecessary costs." As will be discussed in more detail later in this chapter, this has been confirmed by the nonpartisan Congressional Budget Office.

He went on to explain that he has instructed Health and Human Services Secretary Kathleen Sebelius to move forward with "demonstration projects" in certain states. He rightly acknowledged this initiative was first raised by the Bush administration but ultimately turned down by Democrats.

For me, this is not enough—not even close. President Obama had a unique opportunity. He could have put his foot down and said he was going to rein in trial lawyers and hit the reset button. Instead, he offered demonstration projects. What will be gained? The administration will set up a demonstration project in an attempt to show bipartisanship. In the end, it's simply a waste of time. There will be three years of trials, and likely the statistics will not be substantiated. Then, they will call for another three years of study. Too often this is how it works in Washington.

While President Obama understands that malpractice liability reform is needed, it doesn't appear that much will be done about it. Massachusetts Senator John Kerry, whose now discredited 2004 vice presidential running mate John Edwards was a trial lawyer, appeared on *This Week with George Stephanopoulos*. Utah's Republican Senator Orrin Hatch was also a guest.

When the subject of tort reform was raised, Hatch said, "You know, Democrats have been unwilling to take on the personal injury lawyers. And look, there are cases that really deserve awards, huge judgments, but we've got to find some way of getting rid of the frivolous cases, and most of them are."

To his statement, Kerry responded, "And that's doable, most definitely."

We need a uniform, national solution to the problem. It is time for this country to develop a plan that limits frivolous lawsuits, sets up a system to pay economic damages and sets caps on the noneconomic and the punitive portions of malpractice awards.

DEMONSTRATION PROJECTS

Over the past several years, 28 states, to varying degrees, have imposed their own plans to restrain malpractice liability awards. If the Obama administration seeks demonstration projects, they should save taxpayer money and take note of California's Medical Injury Compensation Reform Act, which was discussed in Chapter 2. This "demonstration project" has been successfully underway for the last 34 years. In short, doctors' insurance rates have gone down and patient care has increased. There is voluminous documented proof.

If we look to Texas, we see that tort reform has worked there, too. The Lone Star State enacted malpractice reform legislation in 1995. Since then, physicians have seen their malpractice insurance rates drop significantly.

In 2008, the Perryman Group released a report entitled "The Texas Turnaround." Among its findings, the total impact of tort reforms implemented since 1995 included an annual increase of $112.5 billion in spending each year, as well as approximately 499,900 jobs created in the state. The fiscal stimulus from judicial reforms represents roughly a $2.6 billion per year increase in state tax revenue.

An added benefit was that the reform led to approximately 430,000 individuals having health insurance who would have otherwise gone without it, a result of lowered premiums. With liability insurance savings realized, the Texas Hospital Association said it was able to expand charity care by 24 percent.

Building on the success of the 1995 bill, the Omnibus Tort Reform Bill HB 4 was brought forth by former state Representative Joseph Nixon in 2002, as major reform was still required. "In this backdrop of an effort to provide plaintiffs' remedies for their alleged injuries, Texans were being sued with a greater frequency and ferocity," Nixon stated on behalf of the Texas Public Policy Center. "Doctors were an easy target because they either had insurance or assets necessary to satisfy a judgment." He continued, "Doctors were caught between rising medical malpractice insurance costs and lower compensation from insurance-provided benefit contracts and low Medicare/Medicaid reimbursement levels. Combined with increasing hassles and demands to appear in court or at depositions, doctors were opting to retire or leave Texas." In doctor-per-citizen ratio, he noted, Texas then ranked 48th out of 50 states.

Of Texas' 254 counties, more than 150 had no obstetricians in 2003, and more than 120 had no pediatricians. Five years after the 2003 proposition passed, approximately 7,000 doctors had entered the state, and the State Licensing Board anticipated adding another 5,000 doctors in the coming two years. *The Wall Street Journal* touted the progressive initiative as "Ten Gallon Tort Reform."

A 2008 survey by the Texas Medical Association showed

that 90 percent of physicians in the state said they were more comfortable practicing medicine in Texas now than they were before tort reform was enacted.

In addition, the Texas survey showed that since reform went into effect, the number of malpractice lawsuits has declined; physicians are able to purchase new equipment and can expand the procedures they offer. Further, physicians are more willing to treat high-risk patients. The results in Texas clearly demonstrate that medical malpractice reform does work. I know this to be accurate because we operate facilities in Texas. To me, this is a no-brainer.

TEXAS TORT REFORM

Before Reform: In 2003, a shortage of more than 150 obstetricians and 120 pediatricians existed.

After Reform: Within five years, 7,000 new doctors entered the state. Number of malpractice lawsuits filed dropped by 41%.

While reforms in these states have produced positive results, neighboring states that have not enacted reform continue to suffer. Physicians from states without malpractice reform have often abandoned or limited their practices or simply moved to states with lower rates for malpractice insurance. In either case, the result is that residents of states that have not enacted tort reform have fewer physicians to provide treatment and higher expenses for their healthcare.

A common argument from trial lawyers and others opposed to reform is that the possibility of large jury awards acts as an incentive for doctors to provide better quality care and avoid medical errors. Experience has shown that is not the case, as the incidence of malpractice has not increased in states that have enacted reform.

A 2006 study by *The New England Journal of Medicine* showed that in 25 percent of malpractice lawsuits that resulted in jury awards, there was no identifiable medical error. We do not need more "demonstration projects" to show us that tort reform works. What we need is substantive tort reform.

FEARING LAWSUITS

The American Academy of Orthopedic Surgeons released a report in 2008 by Daniel P. Kessler and Mark B. McClellan that found that one-half of all neurosurgeons—as well as one-third of all orthopedic surgeons, one-third of all emergency physicians, and one-third of all trauma surgeons—are sued each year. As a consequence, 70 percent of emergency departments lack available on-call specialist coverage.

It comes as no surprise that the study also found that 81 percent of responding residents said they view every patient as a potential lawsuit. As a result of excessive, unregulated litigation and waste, it is estimated that this failing system imposes an estimated yearly tort tax of $9,827 for a family of four. In addition, it increases healthcare spending in the United States by an estimated $124 billion: another offshoot of defensive medicine.

In Florida, a medical liability premium for an OB/GYN practicing in Dade County in 2007 was approximately $238,000 per year, which means every time the doctor delivers a baby more than $2,000 goes toward paying the premium.

In states such as California, which enacted limits on jury awards, healthcare costs are between 5 percent and 9 percent less than other states because physicians do not practice defensive medicine.

COST OF LITIGATION

It is estimated that 10 cents of every dollar you spend while visiting your doctor is allocated to malpractice insurance. A practicing doctor with 15 years experience and no record of malpractice is not rewarded; he or she pays the same amount. While malpractice insurance rates for doctors vary from state to state, those states without any reform become prohibitively expensive in which to operate.

Too often trial lawyers will paint the picture that a malpractice suit is essentially a big company with deep pockets going against a poor, wronged individual. Again, if a hospital or doctor is found to be at fault, I support fair and reasonable economic damages but with a cap of $250,000 for noneconomic damages. I would advocate the utilization of annuities or periodic payments as an option for payment for future economic damages, opposed to a lump sum. Additionally, periodic payments are a way to appropriately and rationally compensate the injured as opposed to merely their attorney.

In many states, lawyers have free rein. Regardless of where the alleged malpractice took place, lawyers will almost always venue shop. By and large, they take their cases to inner cities where statistics show that juries favor the individual against the corporation, hospital or doctor, regardless of guilt.

When reform is passed, trial lawyers flee and doctors return. In Texas, for example, Harris County, which covers Houston's courts, found that the number of medical malpractice cases filed in 2005 was down 41 percent from the average number of filings during the six years before 2003. There was a rush in 2003 to file before the new law was enacted, which spiked that year's number to 1,203. The following year, only 204 cases were filed, and that number rose only slightly in 2005 to 256.

Further evidence comes from the University of Texas' System Professional Medical Liability Plan, which insures more than 10,000 physicians and medical students at its six medical centers throughout the state. It released a report citing a 55 percent decline in new lawsuits filed when comparing 2002 to 2005.

As these lawyers enter new fields of litigation, one has to wonder if they were representing the patients because they believed in the claim, or if they were in it for the financial gain. I think the latter.

IT'S TIME TO DO THE RIGHT THING

The Congressional Budget Office reported in 2006 that states with limits on malpractice awards in 1986 saw health care spending per person decline steadily through 2000, ultimately reaching lower levels than in states without caps. Nationwide malpractice reform is not only necessary but beneficial on numerous levels to the operation and administering of health care.

Among states that have realized benefits after taking appropriate action on tort reform is Missouri, which capped noneconomic damages at $350,000. While the legislation was signed into law on 2005, two years prior the eastern portion of Jackson County, one of the state's largest counties, lost its only neurosurgeons due to high malpractice insurance costs. In other areas of the state, there was a shortage of OB/GYNs.

The legislation also derailed venue shopping. As a result, malpractice insurers began turning profits, which opened the door for new insurance companies to write policies in Missouri—real competition. In certain areas of the state, insurance premiums for doctors have dropped by as much as 30 percent, which has resulted in more doctors practicing in the state.

Missouri is among the few states that releases annual statistics on malpractice claims. From 2005 and 2006, average awards in the state declined by 15.9 percent, from $253,888 to $213,454, and by an additional 8.5 percent to $195,239 in 2007.

Due to reform Missouri was able to cut taxes, which in part led to the creation of 70,000 new jobs. Certain legislators are seemingly turning a blind eye to the great strides being made by states that have passed tort reform.

IMPACT ON DOCTOR'S INSURANCE PREMIUMS

In 2008, the Medical Liability Monitor released a report that demonstrated the cost of practicing medicine in different states. Internists in Florida, for example, paid an average malpractice insurance premium of $54,710. In Minnesota, internists paid just $3,375 for similar coverage. In Michigan, a general surgeon paid $143,445, while in South Dakota roughly the same coverage cost $12,569. In New York, obstetricians shelled out $194,935 for insurance while OB/GYNs in Wisconsin paid $18,154.

Trial lawyers are an influential special interest group, and one that seems to prevent the democratic legislators from acting on this issue.

We need to call for a national, federally backed tort reform bill, which should include limiting noneconomic and punitive damages; modifying joint and several liabilities; limit lawyers' fees; establish alternative payment methods for future economic damages; and shorten the statute of limitations on claims. Properly vetting lawsuits is an idea that could positively impact this problem.

Malpractice reform will do more than lower insurance costs for physicians. With federally backed reform in place, doctors could turn their current fixation on costly and unnecessary defensive medicine to focusing their talents and energies on practicing medicine.

Again, the federal government need only look at states like California, Texas and Missouri for a model on which to base a national policy. The groundwork has been laid out for them. A federal solution is needed to avoid the patchwork of laws amongst states, which results in disparate treatment for health care providers and inconsistent availability health care of Americans.

ACCOMPLISHING THE GOAL

President Obama has made it clear that he wants health care reform that will reduce costs, cover the uninsured and not increase the federal deficit. The nonpartisan Congressional Budget Office (CBO) released a report in October 2009 that found that tort reform would cut the federal deficit by $54 billion and reduce health care expenditures by $11 billion. The CBO based it findings upon the elements of tort reform that I am advocating, which states like California have already adopted:

- Capping noneconomic damages at $250,000;
- Capping punitive damages;
- Modifying the collateral source rule;
- Shortening the statute of limitations; and
- Modifying joint and several liability.

Tort reform accomplishes not only President Obama's goals, but also the goals for all Americans that are relative to real and effective health care reform.

Further, President Obama has made it clear that in order to enact health care reform that will benefit all Americans, each of the stakeholders involved in health care must make sacrifices to accomplish the goal. In fact, the hospital industry, of which I am a member, has agreed to absorb and commit $155 billion in losses in order to assist in the goal of universal coverage.

Other stakeholders like the insurance companies, device manufacturers and physicians have also chipped in their financial commitments and agreed to make sacrifices toward this endeavor. Trial lawyers who sue health care providers are a part of this field. However, they have failed and been unwilling to contribute anything out of their pockets while constantly using the health care industry and health care providers as a punching bag for their commercials and closing arguments in the pursuit of contingency fees.

When are the trial lawyers going to kick in? The basic reality of health care reform is that all heath care providers are going to have to do more with less. We are all willing to do this for the betterment of our health care system. How can one expect doctors and hospitals to provide more health care to more people at less cost but still pay expenses and costs in medical malpractice? Fairness and common sense dictate reform, or as Thomas Jefferson said, "Nobody can acquire honor by doing what is wrong."

8

RECOMMENDATIONS ON INSURANCE REFORM

A people that values its privileges
above its principles soon loses both.

– DWIGHT D. EISENHOWER

IF THE FEDERAL GOVERNMENT allowed insurance companies to sell policies across state lines, or in all 50 states, it is estimated that 12 to 14 million of "uninsured" Americans would have the opportunity to access affordable health care insurance. Not unlike enacting national malpractice tort reform, this is another relatively quick solution for a system in need of fixing. Not surprisingly, this particular insurance reform is missing from proposed legislation.

The *American Journal of Medicine* released a study in August 2009 that found in 1981, 8 percent of bankruptcies were attributed to medical bills. In 2001, this figure spiked to 46 percent. In 2007, bankruptcy filings due to medical bills topped 62 percent. There are numerous contributing factors to these staggering figures. However, if Americans are able to shop competitively, select a tailored policy and purchase auto insurance across state lines, why couldn't a similar system be in place for health care insurance?

ALAN B. MILLER

BANKRUPTCIES ATTRIBUTED
TO MEDICAL BILLS

1981: 8%
2001: 46%
2007: 62%

The logical answer: there is no reason why it couldn't happen. One reason it hasn't happened: state bureaucracy. Every state wants to preserve its sovereignty when it comes to the supervision of health insurers. This has little to do with providing health care to the public. It comes down to maintaining a power structure that starts with each state's respective insurance commissioner and filters down to the many departments.

As a result of this system, each state places mandates on what insurance policies should cover—in part the effect of lobbying efforts that are accompanied often with campaign contributions. In the end, the state's administrative fees rise, which in turn raises taxes and health care insurance rates remain overpriced. Is this for the good of the American people?

Once a group of people has the platform to tell a consumer what they should or shouldn't have, the idea of freedom is undermined. With regard to insurance policies, people should have the opportunity to select a policy specific to their needs, age or health status. They should not be excluded for a preexisting condition, a job change or be limited to a few insurance companies.

Instead, we have a system of mandates that serve to

increase premiums and keep more people from obtaining health insurance. For example, a couple in their 50s should not be forced to pay for obstetrical coverage. This approach is counterintuitive.

I'm a businessman and accustomed to taking risk. After a long career, I know that one cannot insure or prepare for every eventuality. Inherently, most people are modest risk takers, too. Americans should be given the choice to decide how much health insurance coverage they want and what deductible they're willing to pay. Every policy has a price or trade-off.

Auto insurance policyholders make a decision—a calculated risk—on what level of coverage, what deductable and premium they are comfortable paying. They understand the consequences. Health care insurance should be no different. To date, the federal government has not had the will to push the envelope and open the market in all states to sales of policies. This, however, has been discussed for many years. A bill was introduced by Representative John Shadegg of Arizona in 2005 intended to do just that. It did not receive enough support. For me, this is a simple solution, and tends to reduce, not increase, costs and serves to make policies affordable to many more people.

AMERICAN BUSINESS: CAPITALISM

Every American should have an equal chance on a level playing field. We need to do a better job at making the health care insurance system fair and open, too. Increased competition gives people many more choices. The market will adapt and respond to an opportunity for increased sales.

If a person is dirt poor, or even reasonably poor, he has Medicaid for coverage. Is it the best program? Perhaps not, but it is access to good health care. Congress should first concentrate on fixing the existing problems before moving forward with any new plans or a massive overhaul of the entire system. There are some who question whether private sector companies should make a profit in the health care field, or if it should be an entirely government run system. In the hospital sector UHS is growing because doctors bring their patients in to obtain high quality health care. And we bring substantial amounts of capitol to the industry. Clearly, for-profit hospitals are a benefit to the system.

Under single-payer health care, competition within the insurance industry will dwindle, and employers will force their folks into the cheaper government plan. The president said everyone can keep their current plan, and no one would be required to enroll in the national plan. True, at the onset, but if it costs $12,000 to cover a family of four and the government is offering the same plan at $6,000 or $7,000, why wouldn't a smart businessperson take that option?

I've spoken to a number of people who run both large and small companies. They said if they have an opportunity to reduce their insurance expenses, they would move their people over to government insurance, and I wouldn't blame them. It makes sense, but only in the short run.

Another provision in the proposed bills would have employers and individuals fined for not providing insurance. When I was working in advertising in New York City in the 1960s, parking my car in the garage would cost around $15. The cost for a parking ticket was around $10, so I often took my chances (but never parked at a fire hydrant). If a business owner is faced with the decision whether to pay $12,000 for an employee insurance policy or receive a lesser cost fine from the government, many will likely pay the fine and come out ahead. And if an individual is fined a few hundred dollars, which is in the recent October 2009 proposal, many will pay the fine and forgo coverage. This is not the solution. In the end, mandating insurance with fines, unless painfully high, will not accomplish the initial goal, which is to ensure every person has an insurance policy.

Single-payer is cloaked under the term of a public option. The option will likely last for a short period of time, then the people covered by private insurance will move into the public option government plan because it will be more attractively priced. At that point, the insurance companies will be hard pressed to remain viable. Does this foster competition? No. It eliminates competition.

As noted previously, the state of Tennessee and its TennCare model should be studied. The program continues to fail. Many business owners took the option and dropped private employee health care policies because they could. This approach serves the lowest common denominator. It is not the American way of tackling a problem.

This is the time to fight the good fight and not succumb to rhetoric and empty promises. A public option could very well be the beginning of the end for this country's superior health care, destroying our system and at an unconscionable cost.

AMERICAN BUSINESS: NEGOTIATION

I'm not in the insurance business, but my company has to

negotiate with insurance companies in regional markets all the time. It is how we do business. While we have locations all over the nation, my business is largely a local, regional business. Others in the same field years ago thought it was best to have a national brand and go across the country and trade on that brand. They found that not to be the best path and it is no longer done. I believed the local hospital was more desirable than a nationally branded one.

Our competition is other hospitals such as a Catholic St. Rose or a nonprofit community hospital. We are generally not in major cities and our competition is usually only two, three or four other hospitals.

Our strategy is to attain the number one or two position in the market. It's a two-fold approach. First we provide high quality health care that will attract doctors. Second, doctors in turn will refer patients. Using this model, we can effectively negotiate with insurance companies. If we only had a small percent share of a given market, the insurance company would propose rates that wouldn't make sense, unreasonable from a cost analysis basis. However, if we have a large enough share of the market, we then have leverage and a fair negotiation can take place. If they do not offer reasonable rates, we play hardball and tell them that we will refuse to take their insurance contract and their clients. So when their non-contracted policyholders come to the emergency room for care, we charge them the non-contract full price.

The negotiated rate is usually well below the full charge rate. Sometimes negotiations are adversarial, but that is how "arms length" business is conducted. They need us and we need them. In the end, by and large, we reach terms that satisfy our needs, and the insurance companies' needs are also met. The cost of the care we provide is efficient and what people receive for their paid premiums is excellent care.

It is estimated that four out 10 Americans who are currently uninsured make $50,000 or more per year. The people in this demographic who are uninsured are not without means. They more likely are people who lost their jobs, are in-between jobs or are on Cobra (extended insurance coverage). They also may be small business owners.

Small business owners and individuals have no clout when negotiating health insurance rates. Premiums are high and some people are forced to go without coverage. If they were allowed to band together into a sizeable group, a fair negotiation would occur with insurers. It would be the same approach as a person shopping auto insurance and deciding between Geico and All State, for example.

A health insurance model would be created that works because enough people would exist in a group to make it profitable for an insurance company to sell a cost effective, affordable policy. The individual and small business owner could select exactly what type of coverage they want, from bare bones to 100 percent coverage.

If the gates were opened and insurance was available across state lines, we would see a niche block of individual business owners and workers banning together to negotiate policies or insurers selling policies at rates to attract these groups.

Presently, individuals can't afford adequate insurance for themselves and their families or offer insurance opportunities to a small group of employees. The idea is to aggregate small business owners such as contractors, storeowners, etc. to able to negotiate and be attractive as a group to insurers.

HEALTH SPENDING ACCOUNTS

This is a different generation. People don't work at one company for 40 years, receive their gold watch and retire. This gives rise to the need for insurance portability.

Instead of employers owning a health insurance policy for employees, let's put ownership of the policy in the hands of the employee. By doing so, coverage would not end with the person's employment but would be taken with the employee when he or she changes jobs. Under this premise, a person changing jobs could not lose coverage due to a technicality such as a preexisting condition or a recent health issue. Everyone seems to agree on this aspect of reform. The insurers have contingently agreed, too.

Payment for the policies could be through Health Spending Accounts (HSA), a program established by the Bush administration. I'm not sure why this concept wasn't promoted more to the American public. It's a terrific idea with no downside.

Nobody spends your money better than you. These accounts were designed to be carried over from year to year. People should have affordable policies and own their insurance. Employer-provided insurance should be personal, decoupled from employment.

Employers and individuals could make contributions to an individual's HSA and that money would be used by the individual to pay for insurance premiums or other health care.

Because the money in the HSA belongs to the individual, there would be more incentive for him or her to spend that money wisely, rather than consume healthcare with little regard to expense.

The initial round of health care reform bills were pushed fast, but the American people, in their wisdom, made it slow down; it wasn't just certain politicians. People are in the process of educating themselves, asking questions and voicing their concerns. This demonstrates that a new level of understanding is being infused into the health care reform debate. The outcome of this issue is tied to our economy, how much we pay in taxes and ultimately how we live. So, people should fully understand what it is they are being asked to support. The stakes are simply too high to ignore.

People will have to better prepare for their future, which includes taking better care of themselves, which makes the HSA program worthy of attention. Counting on the government is a scary proposition. If Americans thought they could retire on Social Security for example, they are sadly mistaken.

SOCIAL SECURITY

When the Social Security Act was passed in 1935 as part of the New Deal, it was sold as a pay-as-you-go program. However, due to medical advances, life expectancy has increased. Now most people are living well past the age of 65, and hence collecting more Social Security benefits.

According to the Social Security Reform Center, in 1950 each retiree's modest benefit was supported by 16 workers, which kept taxes low. Today, that figure has dropped to 3.3

workers per retiree. By 2025, it will equate to approximately two workers per retiree. For the government to continue to pay promised Social Security benefits, taxes must rise or other government services must be cut. The liability here is tremendous.

This year, an estimated 37 million seniors will receive Social Security benefits. According to the Senior Citizens League, 70 percent of beneficiaries depend on Social Security for 50 percent or more of their income. For 15 percent of beneficiaries, Social Security is the sole source of income.

When combined, Social Security and Medicare will absorb an estimated 60 percent of all income taxes collected by 2040. How can the government possibly survive this level of entitlement? If a $1 trillion health care bill is added to this mix, the government in the not so distant future will have to, in addition to raising taxes, choose to support either Medicare, Medicaid or the SCHIP program. There won't be revenue for all.

When approaching the concept of government health care, we must take a good look at the unfunded liabilities that have been created to date.

MANDATORY HEALTH INSURANCE

Overall, it would be desirable if everyone was covered by insurance. The question is how would it be implemented and is mandated insurance constitutional? In the heated Democratic Presidential primary of 2008, Hillary Clinton's position was mandatory insurance for all. The argument was that you need insurance for a car, why not for your health?

Young people, such as those ages 18 to 29, often do not see a need to have it. This is the "invincible" demographic previously noted.

Since insurance companies have fewer healthy people covered by their policies, it increases rates for those who do have insurance. While requiring everyone to have health insurance is a sound principle, there are questions about how it would be enforced and what the penalties would be for those who ignored such a requirement.

According to a Gallup Poll (September 2009), those in the 18 to 34 demographic were split evenly as to whether Congress should vote for or against a health care overhaul (34 percent to 34 percent) while undecided were close behind (31 percent).

TAX CREDITS

Under current laws, people who receive insurance through their employers get a tax-free benefit, while those who have to purchase it on their own have to use after-tax dollars and receive no benefit. This is just not fair. People who purchase plans on their own should receive a tax credit equal to part or all of their coverage, and they should receive a refund when they file their tax returns in April of each year.

This approach, like the many I have outlined, wouldn't be prohibitively expensive. In the end, more people would be insured. They would be better able to buy the insurance that they want and need.

There are other areas where the current administration has made progress, such as the initiative for the health industry to go paperless. As long as privacy issues are addressed, it's a good idea that will increase efficiency, and likely improve health care across the board by reducing medical error. But it will not save a great deal of money for the $2 trillion industry.

The bill called "A New Era of Responsibility: Renewing America's Promise" allocated $630 billion over the next 10 years to finance fundamental reform of our healthcare system. It is intended to bring down costs and expand coverage. Specifically, over the next 10 years, $76.8 billion has been earmarked for technology and innovation. It has been estimated, however, that to transition healthcare facilities to paperless systems could cost $75 billion to $100 billion.

Here again, we have a good idea and initiative; however, if it exceeds the allocated dollar amount, it becomes a money-losing proposition for the government—that money will have to come from somewhere, so little efficiency will have been attained.

LESSONS FROM THE FIELD

I recently obtained a signed photograph of Dwight D. Eisenhower while he was stationed in North Africa in 1943. Not long after the photograph was taken, Eisenhower was surprisingly named to lead U.S. forces in the offensive against Germany.

What a mission! Defeating Hitler's Germany! Eisenhower's bosses, President Franklin Roosevelt and Chief of Staff George Marshall, were eager to start the offensive in Europe in 1943; the wiser and more seasoned Winston Churchill suggested an invasion of North Africa instead. He felt the American army was wet behind the ears and not yet in sufficient number to take on the formidable Germany army. As a result, Eisenhower was placed in charge of Allied forces in North Africa while Churchill built base camps throughout England to accept increasing numbers of American soldiers, supplies and weapons.

After months of preparation, on June 6, 1944, nearly 196,000 heroic soldiers stormed the beaches of Normandy by way of the English Channel.

This decision to place Eisenhower in charge was a disappointment to General Marshall who expressed to President Roosevelt that he wanted the job, as did U.K. General Bernard Montgomery who after success in North Africa made the same plea to Churchill. For Roosevelt's part, he said he couldn't sleep if Marshall were not in Washington. The overall command ultimately given to Eisenhower caused a great rift with Montgomery for the rest of the war.

In the mid 1980s, I took a trip to visit World War II battlefields with veterans of the war. We attended a moving ceremony on June 6 at Normandy and the cemetery above. Then First Lady Nancy Reagan gave a stirring speech remembering the brave soldiers who lost their lives and are buried there.

As our tour continued, we drove through picturesque little towns that were once war-torn. I recall seeing old French soldiers stand proudly at attention, displaying service medals. Many of them had tears in their eyes. It seemed clear they hadn't forgotten the sacrifices America made on their behalf.

I was accompanied on the trip by a then somewhat unknown author, Stephen Ambrose, a professor at the University of New Orleans who was the biographer of Dwight D. Eisenhower and Richard M. Nixon. I came to fully appreciate General Eisenhower during that journey.

As is always the case, there are lessons to be learned from our past. Churchill was wise enough to know that in 1943 the United States wasn't ready to tackle the main objective because equipment, men and supplies had not yet been sent in adequate quantity. But he knew that smaller battles could be won and experience gained.

We are at a crossroads today with regard to health care and, in particular, insurance reform. Why not tackle the manageable aspects of the issue, the problems we know we are able to address and improve rather than overhaul the whole system through a public option.

9

KNOWLEDGE IS POWER

*I don't think much of a man who is not
wiser today than he was yesterday.*

– ABRAHAM LINCOLN

THIS COUNTRY IS CURRENTLY faced with significant problems. The health care reform debate ranks only second to concerns over the economy and the high level of unemployment. In some respects, these two issues are intertwined. In the final analysis, I'm an optimist on both counts.

When you're a businessman, an entrepreneur, you must remain optimistic because the nature of business, like life, is that you will run into problems. My mother was that way—a positive thinker. We had a lot of financial struggles, from making ends meet to caring for my father who had health issues. I never saw her get down on herself or the situation we were in. She was a "can do" type of person. This attitude can be applied to the broken elements of the health care system.

As I said from the beginning, the health care vehicle has broken down. If we simply fix it by applying my recommendations, we won't have to cash in a perfectly viable vehicle just because the current administration sees it as a clunker.

Now, I understand and appreciate that there are many

people on the other side of the debate who also have a "can do" attitude. On some of the major points we agree, such as the concept that insurance companies should not turn away patients because of preexisting conditions or drop sick policyholders when they switch jobs. Insurance should be owned by the individual and sold across state lines. Additionally, a reasonable basic national insurance policy should be framed after detailed study and analysis. HSA, too, should be fostered.

Malpractice tort reform on a national level is essential to meaningful health care reform. Federal regulation will level the playing field for doctors and allow them to practice freely in the state of their choosing. It will also save time and money by putting an end to defensive medicine and have a positive effect that will trickle down through the industry.

Immigration is an overarching issue that impacts many aspects of our society. In the last presidential election it was barely debated because other issues, such as the war in Iraq and Afghanistan, became the focal point.

As a businessman, I'm left to deal with the immigration issue and its influence on our operations. People vote with their feet. Even foreigners that illegally enter the country when in need of health care will opt for the leading hospital. They seek out those facilities that stay ahead of competition. While there are other hospitals in the areas we serve in border towns, illegal aliens go to the hospital where the think they are going to get better care, better equipment, better technicians, better physicians and ultimately a better hospital experience. We see this influx often, and we have to pay for it. This is an unfair consequence resulting from out of control illegal immigration. While hospitals subsidize this group, the American public pays the price too because this raises the cost of care for those with insurance.

SAY NO TO THE PUBLIC OPTION

My intention isn't to bury any aspect of the health care industry. Hypothetically speaking, if the government option was passed, the first couple of years (beginning in 2013) would likely be adequate and wouldn't be bad for my own business.

However, the escalating costs once the program is in place would force the government to realize that they have too many patients and not enough money to support the public insurance plan and Medicare, Medicaid and SCHIP. The government would be forced to cut hospital and doctor fees and institute some form of rationing. What happens next? We would end up like the U.K.: waiting lines increasing exponentially, restrictions on prescriptions of pharmaceuticals, a lack of funding resulting in less innovation and state-of-the art equipment, health care procedures subjected to federally appointed oversight committees and the list goes on.

As a result, people who are in the position to purchase the private health care insurance that remains available will do so. A class system would develop with two tiers of care and ultimately a less healthy nation. Avoiding this nightmare requires a big picture approach: foresight followed by action.

If the public option came to pass, it wouldn't just impact hospitals, doctors and patients, but it would be a major negative for the United States. My career as a businessman has been productive and successful, for which I'm grateful. And while I'm closer to the end of my career than to the beginning, I can't help but feel that the direction we are headed is bad for this generation and generations yet to come.

Under a public option, I fear that the United States will ultimately operate a shabby, underfunded health care system with hospitals that don't have the latest equipment and are mired in bureaucracy.

President Obama perhaps made the best point to support my position on the public option when he told a crowd in August 2009 this: "If the private insurance companies are providing a good bargain and if the public option has to be self-sustaining... I think private insurers should be able to compete. They do it all the time. I mean, if you think about— if you think about it, UPS and FedEx are doing just fine, right? No, they are. It's the U.S. Post Office that's always having problems."

I nearly fell out of my chair when he said those words. It is contradictory. While he might speak well and have a great smile, this unscripted moment underscores that he is unsure of his own platform but conversely understands the private sector's historical strength when competing against government programs. A president that doesn't instill confidence can quickly instill fear. If I had the opportunity to speak to the president, I would tell him how I feel about this all-important health care issue and where I think he is getting it wrong.

Former Vermont governor Howard Dean, who formerly served as the chairman of the Democratic National Committee, said the following statement on MSNBC in August 2009, "The Republican Party is just determined to undermine President Obama, and unfortunately, you have to undermine the country in order to undermine the president and I think that's too bad." This equates to telling the American people that disagreeing with the president is unpatriotic.

At a town hall meeting the following day where he was scheduled to speak in support of the need for a public option, Dean denied saying the above statement on camera. "I did not say that," he said twice and stormed off. He lied and was caught on tape. People watching this debate consider it important and are saying, "Wait just a minute. You're moving too fast."

Aren't we still allowed to disagree with authority in America? This is the very principle our free country was founded upon. If a firm stand is not taken today, then ask yourself where the country will be in five, 10 or 20 years in relation to health care. Interestingly, many of the provisions in the proposed health care bills would not be enacted for three to four years. Is this the same plan that is so urgently needed?

Historically, socialized health care has slowly entered our system. As noted, it began in 1965 with Medicare and Medicaid. If the public option is passed, and insurance reform and malpractice reform are not dealt with as I have outlined, the future of the private sector, free choice medicine in the United States will be questionable.

There has been renewed interest in establishing insurance co-ops since the public option has received so much resistance. The latest proposal presented in October 2009 by the Senate Finance Committee would allocate $6 billion to initiate this effort. Conceptually, these regional co-ops would negotiate contracts with doctors, hospitals and other local providers. Co-ops were first introduced in the 1930s and 1940s before employer-provided insurance tax incentives were passed, which made the approach antiquated. In the current debate, many consider this co-op approach a step backward and a strike against the insurance industry again, which would be forced to compete against government-funded organizations.

The problem with these federally mandated and operated programs is that, at inception, they are considered relatively small or manageable, but within the bureaucratic system, the program grows and grows and the government is obligated to fund it regardless of viability. Take Medicare, which has had a significant number of amendments over the last 40 plus years, all of which called for more coverage—more funding.

It can not be underestimated how difficult it is to establish and then operate a huge, multistate insurance company of magnitude. Some of the nation's leading companies have been in existence for 100 years or more. They have built over time a team of proficient actuaries and policymakers who were trained to understand how to identify risk and set premiums for all sort of groups and individuals in varying circumstances. The federal government is not equipped to successfully operate a program of such magnitude.

YOU HAVE A VOICE

I suggest contacting your representatives and voicing your

concerns on any issues that were raised in this book. A politicians major concern is staying in office. With the 2010 midterm elections around the corner, now is the time to hold your representatives to doing the right thing for America.

If they are not supplying the answers to your questions (doesn't matter if he or she is an incumbent), investigate the other candidate. But if you think they don't make the right decisions, regardless of party, give the other candidate a chance.

And lest we forget, all those in Congress are afforded some of the best health care policies under the Federal Employees Health Benefits Program (FEHBP). These same politicians, who do not face health care coverage issues like the majority of Americans, are in charge of deciding the future direction of our nation's overarching health care policies.

They have an assortment of health plans to select from including fee-for-service, point-of-service and health maintenance organizations (HMOs). In addition, members of Congress are provided the ability to insure their spouses and their dependents. The government pays up to 75 percent of the premium. In short, we, the taxpayers, are footing the health insurance bill for many of the same politicians who are considering derailing our health care system. If we were to ask them if they would join the public plan they propose for America or keep FEHBP, they would likely choose their current plan.

I'll say it again, I'm an optimist. This health care debate has opened the lines of communication. Americans are energized and becoming more informed on the issue with each passing day.

If your state doesn't currently have in place some sort of malpractice tort reform limiting noneconomic damages, ask your representative why and where he or she stands on passage of such a national law. Same goes for insurance reform. Ask them how many insurance companies are allowed to operate in your state. The chances are they can count the number of companies on one hand with one or two enjoying the majority share. Demand more competition.

Talk to your representatives about public option or single-payer system, however it might be phrased. Remember the model of failing programs like Tennessee's TennCare. What looks good on paper doesn't always translate to reality. Who ends up paying? The taxpayer.

Even without a single-payer system, Medicare and Social Security will comprise 60 percent of all federal tax dollars by 2040. We do not need a crystal ball to see the future. We can act now and forego further fiscal crisis. There is no other choice as I see it.

Dialogue between friends, family, coworkers and political representatives is critical to the continuation of this important conversation. It's fine to disagree, but make sure the facts are presented so your informed positions can be supported.

After all, we are talking about our collective health and welfare as well as the prosperity and longevity of these United States of America. A great nation, blessed by God.

THE MAN BEHIND
UNIVERSAL HEALTH SERVICES, ALAN B. MILLER

LARRY B. PULLEY,
Dean of the Mason School of Business, The College of William & Mary

Success is not final, failure is not fatal;
it is courage to continue that counts.

– WINSTON CHURCHILL

PERHAPS ALAN B. MILLER'S SUCCESS is summed up by his own business philosophy: "One basic lesson I learned and always practice is leading by example. People will follow you if they believe and trust in you, put their future in your hands, but without trust you can't be an effective leader."

To date, more than 38,000 people follow Miller as the Chairman and Chief Executive Officer of Universal Health Services, Inc. (UHS), a leading hospital management company that owns and operates acute care hospitals, behavioral health centers, ambulatory surgery centers and radiation oncology centers.

In total, UHS, which celebrates its 30th anniversary in 2009, owns 137 hospitals in 32 states and Puerto Rico with annual revenues exceeding $5 billion. This is quite a hop, skip and a jump from the working class neighborhood in Crown Heights, Brooklyn, where Miller was born.

When not playing stickball or baseball, Miller was an industrious youngster, working after-school jobs as a delivery clerk for a grocery store and for Western Union. A bright student, he skipped a grade, managed to excel in advanced placement courses and graduated high school at age 16.

Miller's parents were hardworking, second-generation Americans from a Russian immigrant background. His father owned a dry cleaner store and his mother worked for a millinery company. "My mother was smart, strong willed and had a strong personality. This is where I likely got my leadership qualities from because I'm also strong willed," said Miller. "My mother was the dominant one in the family until my father got annoyed," Miller added with a laugh. "My father was thoughtful and compassionate, so there was a balance."

Standing six foot five inches tall, Miller's aptitude and love for the game of basketball scored him a full scholarship to the then top ranked University of Utah, but not before helping to lead his high school team to victory in the New York City championship in 1954, an undefeated season.

"That championship experience is an example of how endless hours of practice and teaming up with others with talent can lead to success," said Miller. "I had red hair and a temper, so in high school they gave me the nickname 'Red,'" Miller said with a laugh.

While he was excited to experience life beyond the streets of New York, the University of Utah would lose its grip on Miller. "It was an interesting experience but ultimately the wrong choice for me," he said. Brought to the attention of the College of William and Mary's head basketball coach, Miller, a freshman star, was given a full scholarship, sight unseen.

After only one year of varsity play, tragedy struck while his team was en route to play the University of Pennsylvania. A severe car accident left Miller close to death. He would spend a month in a Washington, D.C. hospital recuperating from a fractured skull and broken jaw. A number of subsequent procedures were required to repair all the damage.

More devastating than the crash, Miller's basketball career unfortunately ended. Miller turned his interests toward attaining knowledge and experience. He graduated the College of William & Mary with a bachelor's degree in economics.

It was the hardship he faced both on and off the court that shaped his approach to reaching his goals. "Athletics teaches you to overcome obstacles and to not give up. There is a parallel to business. It's a question of being dogged and not being discouraged."

A scholarship enabled Miller to attend an out-of-town university, which was important to him. After achieving that goal, he pushed forward and received a Masters in Business Administration from the Wharton School of the University of Pennsylvania. After ROTC, at the William and Mary graduation he received a commission as a lieutenant in the U.S. Army. He later served in the 77th Infantry Division, retiring with the rank of captain.

"To me there are no better people than those who are willing to serve our country in the military," said Miller, who wears an American flag on his lapel in solidarity with U.S. troops fighting in Iraq and Afghanistan.

TIME TO GET COOKING

Miller entered the advertising industry in the early 1960s. His first job was with the Kudner Agency in New York City. Eventfully, he was hired by Young & Rubicam, where he spent most of his eight-year advertising career, quickly excelled, and was eventually named one of the company's youngest vice presidents.

It was during this fertile time period that Miller was exposed to the spirit of entrepreneurship. The rewards that laid in wait for those who took risks excited him. One such project was an account that required working with an unknown chef. Miller became an instrumental force that helped to create the first nationally syndicated television program called *The Galloping Gourmet*, with Graham Kerr.

A NEW DIRECTION

Conversations with Miller's Wharton roommate in 1969 would change the course of his career. An idea was hatched for a new venture: building privately owned hospitals in high growth areas such as California, Nevada, Texas and Florida. Giving into his entrepreneurial spirit, Miller agreed and joined American Medicorp, a pioneering start-up private hospital company.

American Medicorp enjoyed great growth and success until 1973 when financial troubles almost sank the company. Miller's roommate left the company as it was on the brink of insolvency. Miller took the reins becoming CEO. Faced with adversity, he went to work and managed a classic business turnaround.

By 1978, the company was a success and well-positioned

in the market. This gained the attention of the entire health-care industry, but such attention had a downside. The company became the target of a hostile takeover by Humana, Inc. since the price of its publicly traded shares lagged its accomplishments.

While TWA also made a bid for American Medicorp., as well as offered Miller the position of president of the company, it wouldn't be enough to thwart Humana's takeover. Fighting to the end, Miller was able to raise Humana's offer price by double, which generated a handsome payday for shareholders, while Miller chose to leave.

"I learned valuable lessons from that experience," Miller reflected.

The day after Humana's hostile takeover was completed, Miller, ever the optimist, started a new company in the same industry, Universal Health Services, Inc. "The people I started with all came from American Medicorp. So we just went up the street, rented an office, got a telephone and started looking for hospital opportunities."

Started in 1978 with $3.2 million in venture capital and $750,000 of his own money with six employees and zero revenue, Miller, through years of hard work, turned Universal Health Services into a Fortune 500 company.

"Our goal is not to be the biggest provider of healthcare services but the best in the communities we serve," said Miller. "My attitude has been 'can do' positive, even when things have been difficult."

Recognizing his fortitude, the Federation of American Health Systems bestowed on Miller the Award for Leadership in 1978. Twenty-one years later, he would receive the organization's highest honor, the first Lifetime Achievement Award.

Miller further expanded his business interests. In 1986, he founded the Universal Health Realty Income Trust, a real estate investment trust which invests in healthcare related facilities including acute care hospitals, behavioral healthcare facilities, rehabilitation hospitals, subacute care facilities, surgery centers, childcare centers and medical office buildings.

To date, the company has 49 real estate investments in fifteen states. Miller holds a unique distinction in that he is the chairman and chief executive officer simultaneously of two publicly traded companies on the New York Stock Exchange.

"I had the great pleasure of spending an hour with John Wooden, the Hall of Fame basketball player and coach whose UCLA men's team won an unparalleled 10 NCAA Championships in 12 years," said Miller. "I have a signed basketball from him. I have a file of articles about him, because when you find a man who is so successful and who has so much knowledge, you should try and learn from him." And one would be surprised at how fiery he is, since his outward demeanor is gentlemanly and subdued.

PROGRESSIVE PERSEVERANCE

Accolades were bestowed on Miller throughout his career. In 1991, he was named Entrepreneur of the Year, an award sponsored by Ernst & Young and Merrill Lynch. In 1995 and 1996, Miller was listed among the Outstanding 1,000 CEOs in the nation. In the latter year, he served as the Chairman of the Philadelphia United Negro College Fund Corporate Campaign for which he received the Organization's Chairman Award. He was awarded an honorary doctorate from the University of South Carolina. Since 2003, he has been one of *Modern Healthcare* magazine's "100 Most Powerful People in Healthcare." He also is recipient of the George Washington University Medal for his development of the world-class hospital located on its campus.

Miller is humble and reserved, although a quick-witted observation and a hearty laugh are seemingly always moments away. He is both interested and interesting. "I've never asked an employee to do a job I wouldn't do," said Miller. "It would offend my sense of fairness."

A tireless executive, Miller serves on the Board of Directors of The Penn Mutual Life Insurance Company and the Kimmel Performing Arts Center in Philadelphia and as the Chairman Emeritus of the Opera Company of Philadelphia. An ardent supporter of the education of students of varying means, he served on the executive board of the Wharton School of the University of Pennsylvania and the Board of Overseers of the internationally known business school.

Miller is a lifetime member of the College of William & Mary's President's Council and he received the College's highest honor, the William and Mary Medal in 1999. He was a trustee of the College of William & Mary Endowment Fund. In October 2007, the business school awarded him the T.C. and Elizabeth Clarke Business Medal, the school's highest honor for business achievement. Later in 2007, the college announced the creation of the Alan B. Miller Center for Entrepreneurship.

"I was looking to give back to William & Mary for the scholarship I got when I attended school," Miller said. "Anyone can contribute, but you hope you can do it in a way that would be truly helpful. Look, we all want to be supportive; we all want to do good things." He continued, "I love America and I believe that economic power derived from business accomplishments is what has allowed America to be a leader in the world. This school will train young people to be business leaders and to help develop entrepreneurs and they in turn will build prosperous companies that generate jobs. I wanted to be part of that."

The center, along with the entire Mason School of Business at the College of William & Mary, will be housed in the new Alan B. Miller Hall. In honor of his parents, Mary and Manuel, he established scholarships in Liberal Arts and basketball many years ago. He also funded the construction of the gymnasium in the college's state-of-the-art recreation center.

Reflecting on the importance of Miller Hall, he said, "Think about business schools. Highly desirable prospects visit the buildings at colleges; and if they don't see top-rated facilities, they believe that the school is not dedicated to the program," he continued. "If you don't demonstrably invest resources in a program, top-rated prospects will go somewhere else. It happens all the time. Winston Churchill said, 'We shape the building and then they shape us.' How true! First-class facilities elevate everyone involved."

His dedication and service to civic organizations has been recognized throughout the years. In 1992, he was awarded the Ellis Island Medal of Honor in recognition of his "exceptional humanitarian efforts and outstanding contributions to the country" through health care. He is also a past recipient of the Americanism Award from the Anti-Defamation League.

Happily married to his wife Jill for more than 40 years, the couple has two daughters, Marni and Abby, and a son, Marc, a fellow Wharton alumnus and the recently named president of Universal Health Services.

Since founding Universal Health Services, Miller has brought a sense of family to the corporate structure, which has extended to the facilities the company operates.

"We are supportive of the communities that we serve, and they know that we are there when they need us. All of our hospitals are full service, and we are on the front lines when there is an emergency," said Miller. "We believe in supporting the community and being good corporate citizens."

THIRTY YEARS OF EXCELLENCE

"In terms of opportunity, I see it all the same," Miller said of UHS turning 30. "People have often asked, 'Did you ever think your company would grow so big?'" Miller said. "I never thought about it that way. I was always interested in quality and not size. My goal was to have a sterling reputation built on excellence of service, fairly earned. That was, and is, the most important thing to me."

"Being the biggest (company) was never the goal. I wanted to be big enough to attract capable people and provide exceptional services," said Miller. "My goal was to be known as a top-quality company in the industry. I believe, as do many others, that we are the top-quality company in our industry; our record is unique. We have been at it for 30 years. We have always been profitable and have never been involved in scandal, and our strategy has been proved correct over the years."

Among publicly traded hospital operators, UHS has one of the most diversified business (mix) profiles, with substantial earnings generated both from its acute care and behavioral health segments.

More than 350 work at corporate headquarters located in King of Prussia, Pennsylvania. One of the keys to the company's success is loyal, long tenured employees.

"We've put a premium on ethical and fair conduct in business. We attract and retain people who have a conscience, in addition to high competence at their jobs," said Miller.

Miller is known as an accessible CEO, as are his senior executives. Any unnecessary bureaucracy has been stripped from the company's business model, which has streamlined operations. UHS employees agree that Miller is a straight shooter with a big heart.

After the September 11th tragedy, UHS offered to match the contributions employees made to a fund established to assist the families of lost firefighters. Miller personally delivered the sizeable check to the Firefighters Union in New York City. "While others procrastinated, we delivered funds that were needed immediately," he noted.

"One of the things that attracts people to this business and keeps them working enthusiastically is the knowledge that they are contributing to the people in their communities and to society in general," Miller said. "I think we have almost a blessed career path because we're part of a business that is focused on helping people often with serious problems."

Over the course of Miller's career, corporate culture and the way in which business is conducted has changed. The proverbial handshake is no longer binding. But many have done business with him on the basis of promises, and they are always kept.

"The country is on a fast track. A lot of business that was conducted for years and years with people that one knew, financiers or lawyers and the like, has changed. People used to know the character of the person they were dealing with. Long-standing relationships slowly faded, and today, to many, personal relationships don't matter, it is all about the transaction," said Miller.

"For example, we had a long financial relationship with a bank, Continental Illinois of Chicago. This bank took American Medicorp's proprietary information and gave it to Humana, who in turn used this information to take over my company. We believed our relationship with the bank was based on a high degree of ethical behavior as well as legal obligations."

"Today, that bank is gone. Take Lehman Brothers—we had a relationship with them, too. One of its partners did work with us just to get inside information on the company, for that same take over and now they are gone. So, I didn't shed a tear when either one of those companies went away. I believe if you do something unprincipled in one instance that is indicative of how you do business. It's not a one-time thing; you either do that sort of thing or you don't. Ultimately, in these two cases they failed."

THE FUTURE IS BRIGHT

Looking forward, Miller said, "How big UHS will be depends on the opportunities. We will focus on providing quality services. We buy in a disciplined way. We don't have to do deals. When we see an opportunity, we have the financial capability to act, we are in a position to do anything we would want to do, and that's a good position to maintain."

Starting with six employees and zero revenue and building to 38,000 employees and $5 billion in revenues, Miller doesn't rule out the possibility that similar growth and success could be achieved in the next 30 years.

"I don't see why not. I actually think it is easier today because the larger you are the more capabilities you have and the more opportunities you see. But again, I don't think in those terms. I have no idea how large the future Universal Health Services will be. The culture of quality— doing the right thing—hiring good, talented people who understand what we stand for and are concerned about the reputation of the company...these are the enduring values. Whether the company grows to $10 billion or $20 billion, it's immaterial," said Miller.

Universal Health Services is well-positioned moving forward as it has one of the most conservative balance sheets in the industry, providing both financial and operational flexibility. While the majority of the industry operates on high leverage ratios, UHS has a favorable profile; debt, for example, represents only 39 percent of the total capitalization of the company, versus the industry average of 72 percent.

Reflecting on the Humana takeover, Miller said, "Financially I did very well, but that wasn't the point. The company and its reputation were growing, the employees and management were performing well, and then all of sudden, it went away."

"In the end, I had to start all over. I was challenged to utilize all my acumen and capabilities. Looking back 30 years later, it wasn't easy or enjoyable at the very beginning, but it was all worth it."

BIBLIOGRAPHY

"1965 Advisory Council on Social Security—Hospital Insurance for the Elderly and Disabled, Part II." Social Security Online, http://www.ssa.gov/history/reports/65council/65part2.html

"2008 Older Americans: Key Indicators of Well-Being." Federal Interagency Forum on Aging Related Statistics, 2008. http://www.agingstats.gov/agingstatsdotnet/Main_Site/Data/2008_Documents/Population.aspx

Appleby, Julie. "Health Care: Lowering Costs for Old Could Raise Them for Young." USA Today, August 30, 2009. http://www.usatoday.com/money/industries/health/2009-08-30-health-insurance-premiums-debate_N.htm

"The American Medical Association—MSS CTUW Modules Number 3 Health Insurance Statistics." http://www.ama-assn.org/ama1/pub/upload/mm/15/ctuw_module_3.pdf

Bailey, Holly. "Poll Watch: Americans Still Split on Health-Care Reform, Say It Will Affect 2010." Newsweek, September 8, 2009.

Campbell, Paul. "Rockefeller's Proposes a New MedPAC to Focus on Delivery System Reform and Limit CMS' Role in Payment Policy." Health Reform Musings, May 29, 2009. http://www.healthreformmusings.com/2009/05/articles/new-technologies/rockefellers-proposes-a-new-medpac-to-focus-on-delivery-system-reform-and-limit-cms-role-in-payment-policy/

Cannon, Michael. "Massachusetts' Obama-like Reforms Increase Health Costs, Wait Times." Real Clear Politics, September 5, 2009. http://www.realclearpolitics.com/articles/2009/09/05/obamacare_increases_costs_wait_times_98176.html

"CMS Announces Medicare Premiums, Deductibles for 2009." Centers for Medicare & Medicaid Services and U.S. Department of Health and Human Services, 2009. http://www.cms.hhs.gov/apps/media/press/factsheet. asp?counter=3272

"Expanding Health Insurance: The AMA Proposal For Reform." The American Medical Association, Volume 2, 2007.

Fagin, Darryl. "Reform bill complex enough without this low-yield factor." *La Crosse Tribune*, September 1, 2009.

Furchtgott-Roth, Diana. "The High Cost of Medical Malpractice." Reuters, August 6, 2009. http://blogs.reuters.com/great-debate/2009/08/06/ reduce-the-high-cost-of-medical-malpractice/

"The Health Crisis History." PBS, http://www.pbs.org/healthcarecrisis/ history.htm.

"Hospital Adjusted Expenses per Inpatient Day." AHA Annual Survey 2007. http://www.aha.org/aha/research-and-trends/health-and-hospital- trends/2007.html

Jensen, Kristin and Laura Litvan. "Health-Care Plan Future Rests on Snowe, Democrats." Bloomberg, October 12, 2009. http://www.bloomberg.com/ apps/news?pid=newsarchive&sid=aCQK9wFnaZZo

Johnson, Lyndon B. "Statement by the President Following Passage of the Medicare Bill by the Senate—July 9, 1965." Center for Medicare and Medicaid Services, July 9, 1965. http://www.cms.hhs.gov/History/ Downloads/CMSPresidentsSpeeches.pdf

Jones, Terry. "45% Of Doctors Would Consider Quitting If Congress Passes Health Care Overhaul." *Investor's Business Daily*, September 15, 2009.

Kerry, John and Orrin Hatch. *This Week with George Stephanopoulos*. ABC News. August 30, 2009.

Martin, Amy. "Study Shows More People Go Without Health Coverage as Insurance Costs Outpace Income Eight-fold." Cover the Uninsured Project, March 24, 2009. http://covertheuninsured.org/content/study-shows-more-people-go-without-health-coverage-insurance-costs-outpace-income-eight-fold

Martin, Marian. "Fighting For TennCare." *The Jackson Sun*, September 20, 2009.

"Massachusetts Health Care Reform Three Years Later." Kaiser Commission on Medicaid and the Uninsured, September 1, 2009. http://www.kff.org/uninsured/7777.cfm

Meehan, Chris, ed. "New Studies Suggest That Blues Plans Have 'Near-Monopolies' in Some States," *The AIS Report on BlueCross BlueShield Plans*, July 7, 2009. http://www.aishealth.com/Bnow/hbd070709.html

Shadegg, John and Pete Hoekstra. "How to Insure Every American." *The Wall Street Journal*, September 4, 2009.

Stein, Rob. "Is the Mayo Clinic a Model Or a Mirage? Jury Is Still Out." *The Washington Post*, September 20, 2009.

Tasker, Fred. "'Underinsured' Face Challenges Paying for Health Care." *The Miami Herald*, September 3, 2009.

"Texas' Tort Reform Gives Example for Other States." *Tyler Morning Telegraph*, May 27, 2008.

"Underinsured." Consumer Reports, August 6, 2007. http://www.consumeraffairs.com/news04/2007/08/cu_insurance.html

Weinstein, Stuart L. "The Cost of Defensive Medicine." *AAOS Now*, November 2008. http://www.aaos.org/news/aaosnow/nov08/managing7.asp

"Who are the Uninsured?" *The Washington Times*, Editorial. June 25, 2009.